WALKING
MY WAY
BACK TO ME

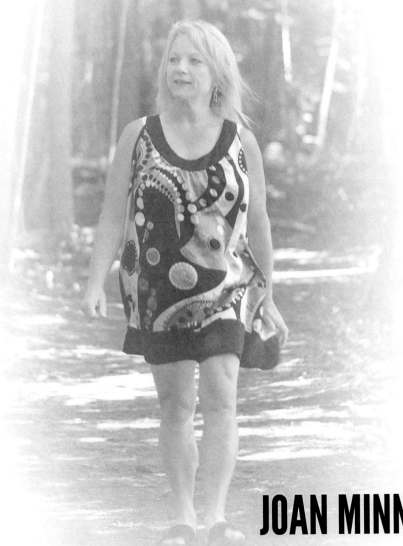

JOAN MINNERY

DISCLAIMER: THIS INFORMATION (AND ANY ACCOMPANYING PRINTED MATERIAL) IS NOT INTENDED TO REPLACE THE ATTENTION OR ADVICE OF A PHYSICIAN OR OTHER HEALTH CARE PROFESSIONAL. ANYONE WHO WISHES TO EMBARK ON ANY DIETARY, HERB, SUPPLEMENT, DRUG, EXERCISE, OR OTHER LIFESTYLE CHANGE INTENDED TO PREVENT OR TREAT A SPECIFIC DISEASE OR CONDITION SHOULD FIRST CONSULT WITH AND SEEK CLEARANCE FROM A QUALIFIED HEALTH CARE PROFESSIONAL.

Joan Minnery Enterprises
117 Morton Avenue
Brantford, ON, Canada N3R2N9

Library and Archives Canada Cataloguing in Publication

Minnery, Joan. 1966

Walking My Way Back To Me / Joan Minnery

ISBN 978-0-9938909-0-1

1. Health. 2. Autobiography 3. Weight Loss 4. Inspiration 5. Self Help

1.   Title

Layout by Ball Media, Brantford ON | www.ballmedia.com
Printed and bound in Canada, First Edition

Dedicated to my son, Bill "BJ" Minnery (the Beej),
whose deepest wish was to be able to
put his arms around his Mama.

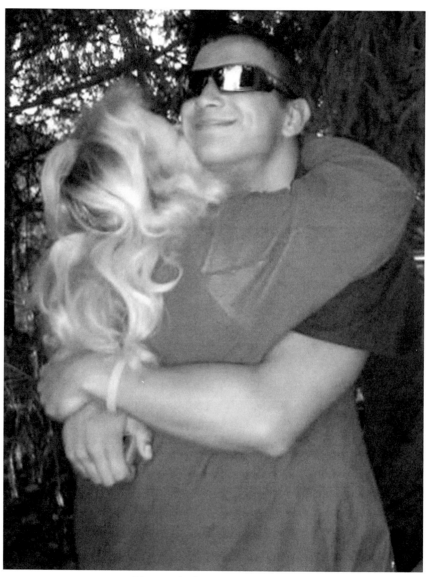

My son's face says it all!!!

FOREWORD Written by Bill Minnery

I don't even think I knew what fat or being fat was until our vacation to Orlando, Florida's Disney World when I was ten years old. Not because Florida is filled with a lot of overweight people, but because when my mom tried to bring the safety bar down over her head, it would not snap into place for her or for me and two other passengers on the Tower of Terror ride. Her oversized belly was actually stopping the bar from snapping all the way down and once the bar did snap down with help from one of the ride's employees it looked like it was prohibiting her from getting full and complete breaths. I looked around at everyone on the ride. They were all staring at my mom like she was a freak of nature. I could hear their thoughts, *"Why would she even get on the ride?"* and *"She's fat."* This was the first time I had ever seen my mom physically and mentally crumble in front of my eyes. My mom tried to compose herself as best as she could, and made it seem like nothing happened. The blood quickly rushed to her face, causing her cheeks to blush red and it instantly gave away her embarrassment. Since I had never witnessed her act like this before, I had no idea how to react to the situation. I stared forward in silence awaiting the start of the ride.

As soon as the ride started and being only ten years old, I completely forgot about the embarrassing situation that just took place and was mesmerized by the ride's illusions, twists and turns. Halfway through the ride, I looked over at my mom and I could tell she was obviously sucking in and probably having trouble breathing. All of a sudden the ride stopped and two massive doors swung open in front of us. We were about 200 feet up overlooking Disney's MGM Studios. A push of hot and humid air flew through the ride and at that moment I realized the ride turned into a drop zone. Out of nowhere, we suddenly dropped for what seemed to be a long time. It then dropped several times over again. My mom had her 260lb diaphragm and belly pressing against the safety bar as her breathing was restricted. I had no idea that this was happening until the ride stopped.

I had the time of my life. My mom, on the other hand, went white as a ghost, was shaking and screaming at the Disney employee to lift up the safety bar because she could not breathe. The bar lifted and instantly I could see the pressure release off of her belly and finally she was able to breathe correctly. She stood up, got off the ride and keeled over, almost falling to her knees gasping for air. I was shocked and apparently so was she. I asked myself, *"Is anyone else seriously affected by this ride?"* I looked around to all of the fellow people and not any of them were physically sick. Why was my mom the only person almost passing out after the ride? The answer was obvious: she was too fat. That was the first moment I realized my mom had any type of physical problem and it was a big one. My mom rushed to the closest garbage can, vomiting in the outside receptacle. She continued to get nauseous for the next day while we were on vacation. From that moment, it was something that seriously bugged me and got on my nerves.

Over the years, I would bring up her eating habits but whenever I did, I would get shut down or an argument would start. I love my mom but I hated her weight. I could see the beauty underneath which she tried so hard to cover up. She had everything going for her except for her weight. I don't even know how many nights I would witness her in the bathroom all night long throwing up and having digestive difficulties because of the types and amount of food she was eating.

Eventually my mom, who is only five foot two inches, skyrocketed to 280lbs. In comparison, Brock Lesnar, a very famous WWE wrester and UFC fighter is six foot three and he's also 280lbs. When you think of it like that, it's crazy. Her heart was pumping over and above what it should have been, 24 hours a day.

When I started high school and started taking health classes I began learning about how unhealthy my mom actually was. If

Walking My Way Back To Me

I look back at memories of my mom from childhood I probably wouldn't be able to picture her without a can of coke in her hand. Chain-drinking Coca-Cola was like her own personal form of smoking. By the time I was eighteen, I had already come to terms with the fact that my mom would probably not be here by the time I was twenty five. I knew that my mom clearly only had years left until life altering problems began. I thought she would die either of a heart attack or gall bladder cancer. On her small frame, nearly 300 pounds on a hobbit of a human is just too much. I began being unable to handle it anymore and snapped on her telling her exactly how I was feeling. *"Mom, I'm eighteen. I love you with all of my heart, but I know for a fact that you won't be here by the time I'm twenty five. You're fat as Hell, you're unhealthy and this is your last chance to become who I know you're meant to be."* I saw my mom's anger but I also saw her sadness. There is only one person in the world who could have said these kinds of things to my mom to whom she would actually listen and it was me. Every person in the world usually has at least one or two people who they trust more than anything. These are the people who can save your life if they choose to get past awkward moments. I chose to get through that awkward moment. To me, it meant everything and eventually it meant that to my mom.

Mom goes into the details of the "A-Ha" moment within the pages of this book, so I'll let her tell that story. What I can say is that once her brain flipped over, it was the beginning of everything. I've witnessed my mom go on too many failed diets. This time there was a certain spark in her face and an attitude that I have never seen before in my life.

During the 'journey,' my mom quit driving everywhere completely, which was great for me, because it meant I got to use the van. She started to lose a considerable amount of weight very quickly, as she was walking everywhere and eating properly. I couldn't have been happier for her because I could tell it was never going to end. Not just because of her attitude, but because she literally took away any aspect of her life that would lead her to food, even sacrificing friends.

Now, 150 pounds later, I can see my mom the way she's

always wanted people to see her. Her body completely used to contradict who she was and now it matches her. All of this would NOT have happened if I decided to avoid being straight up with her about the problems she had. No one ever wants to talk down and pretty much embarrass their mother face-to-face but I am telling you it was the best decision I have made. In my eyes, I saved her by being firm, harsh and truthful. It was love straight from the heart.

My mom is my best friend, always has been since the very beginning and always will be. She has always been by me no matter what, through every single problem I've endured. She deserved my help with her health and weight. If I didn't speak up to my mom and suck it up, who knows what could have happened to her by now. All I know is she is on fire with the journey and happier than I've ever seen her. This is exactly what I wanted for her. My dream for my mom came true. If there is anyone reading this who has someone close to them with a serious weight problem or even just a general problem and you know you are the person for whom they have complete love and trust, speak up because I promise you, in the end, it will be worth it. You can unmistakably begin a series of thoughts for a person which makes them begin their path to a healthy and longer life.

Mom, I love you. Thank you for everything. 117.
@skillbill

INTRODUCTION - IF I CAN DREAM

"I am responsible for the energy I bring into my own space."

A note to my Readers

From the onset of this project, it was my desire to present this story as if my readers and I were sitting on a park bench and chatting. The book had to be informative, yet laid back and in an atmosphere that allowed for easy reading. It was paramount that any messages were conveyed through raw honesty and integrity.

Writing an autobiography is like pulling your own teeth out without any local anesthetic. When you write about yourself, you have to bare your soul. Honesty can be painful. I wanted to write about the steps I had taken to *change my life*, but in order to do that, I needed to *write* about my life. Being honest with oneself is also therapeutic. I knew that my story would help others, and in return, I have also helped myself. Through telling my own story I have been able to look at the roadmap of my own life and truly find myself. I've come to the conclusion that for all of my stories I must take complete ownership of being the author.

Walking My Way Back To Me is a Love Story which I have divided into three parts: *FAT, FIT & FREE.*

"FAT" is the first and longest section is as it depicts my life from childhood until August, 2010. Naturally it is the most detailed as I lived on the larger side of life for over four decades. It is a chronological account of how I functioned as a fat person and ineffectively hid the side effects of a compromised body suffering from self-abuse. "FIT" is the second section, detailing my weight loss journey from August 27, 2010 until March, 2012. It gives the physical, emotional and mental steps that I had to take in order for my journey to happen correctly. "FREE" is the final section of my life from spring of 2012 until summer of 2014. It is the outcome of being free from the bondage I levied upon myself within the confines of my clothing and my much wounded heart. It is about establishing forgiveness. It is about the freedom of my body and the freedom of my mind - both of which were necessary in order for me to move forward. The weight on my body was minuscule compared to the weight on my shoulders. Freedom happened during and after weight loss. It plays a direct impactful step towards healing. My chapter titles are Elvis related and taken from some of his great hits. As he's been my main musical influence and has played the pivotal male lead in my adult life, it is a direct homage to him and fans alike.

My awakening helped me fully understand and finally accept that I had done the damage to my own body. That laying blame was the cloak behind which I hid. My reasons for being fat are not another person's but I am willing to bet there are extreme similarities with my story and any other person battling the bulge. It is within the pages that I wanted to tell my story in order to dispel those myths and reach out to others who like me, have suffered in silence and been the victim of their own self. They need to know that they are not alone. Somebody knows their story and has been candid enough to reach into the deeply personal side. It is OK to break the barrier of taboo topics and stop living in the shadows of the reality we never want to talk about. Perhaps in that admittance, it will bring others forward into their own journey.

I didn't start to be thin. I started because I needed to be healthy, not just physically but mentally. Four decades of self abuse and the burden of a lifetime of ridicule carries a lot more weight than what was on my ankles!!! This was not about vanity, it was about sanity. I had to give myself a chance. I had searched the world for someone to take a chance on me and realized that the person who needed to give me a chance – was me. I was worth it. I was worth taking a chance on.

Walking My Way Back To Me...

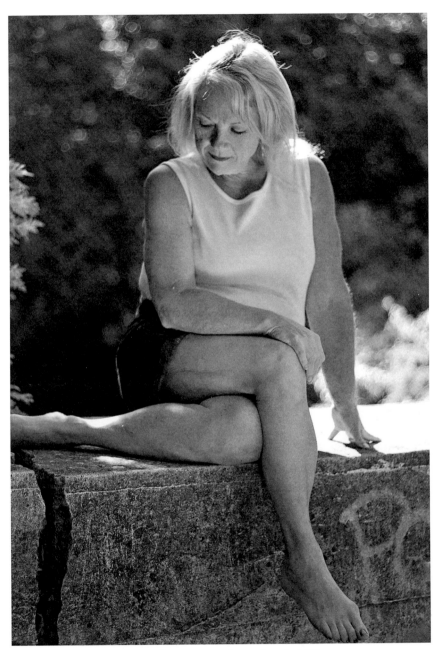

The infamous rock at App's Mill.

Joan Minnery

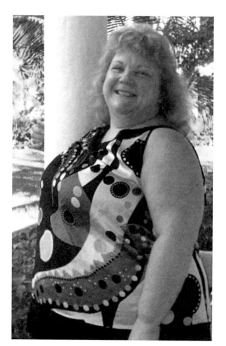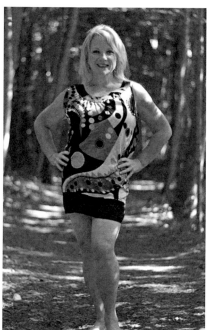

My Journey....

FAT

Every human being is the author
of his own health or disease

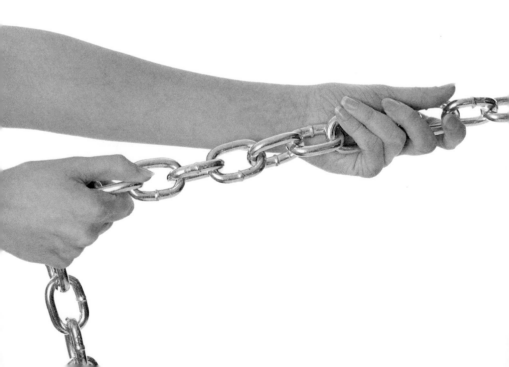

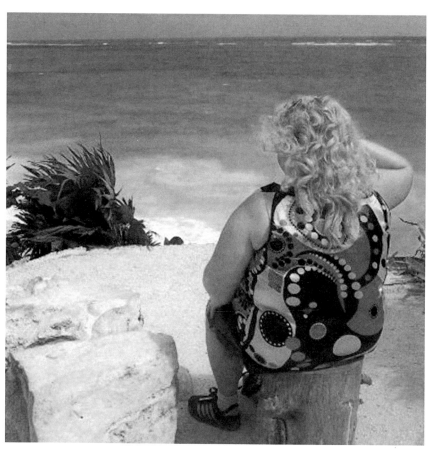

Searching for the answer...

WELCOME TO MY WORLD

Every person has a story. There is an overwhelming, underlying reason why people overeat. It's never about food. It's about a life story. Each of us has a vice and a coping mechanism to deal with our story. Whether it's smoking, taking drugs, drinking alcohol, acting out, or abusing our bodies through gorging, we all do something to deal with our own demons. We could take one hundred overweight people in a room and ask them all the same question and each one of them would have a similar story -- food is not the cause, it's the foundation of losing control and getting in our own way as we have had to deal with our story. We are the authors. We have a simple choice to make: *"Do we write a sob story or a success story?"*

If you are going to write a book about losing weight, teach others how to effectively keep it off and offer weight loss tips, first and foremost, you'd better be an expert on the exact opposite. After spending forty four years overweight, I am a fat expert. I know how to be fat, how to stay fat, how to avoid fat, how to avoid being fat, and how to co-exist with a security blanket around me, which IS fat. I know everything about being a fat person. I lived that life for 99% of my time here on Planet Earth. Standing on the biggest stage I've ever known, in front of the largest audience I will ever face, I proudly say, *"My name is Joan Minnery. I am a food addict and I suffer from gluttony."*

I had been a rotund person all of my life. I was a pudgy child, a husky teen, a large sized adult and morphed into an obese person in my late thirties. On a short petite five foot two frame, I looked like the cousin of the Pillsbury Dough Boy. Add in the platinum

15

hair, the blue eyes and an ample bosom, my small package was oozing. But that's what happens when you continually pour mud into a bag; it eventually bursts.

I have had a love affair with food and the make believe world of Hollywood for all of my years. I was star struck and there was none that shined brighter than Elvis Presley. I too wanted to be a star. There isn't a friend of mine from my younger years who doesn't reminisce about Joan and her Hollywood aspirations. Singing, acting, dancing -- I was going to be famous, a triple threat. My brother John joked that one day they would see me accepting my trophy at the Academy Awards, holding the Oscar in one hand while holding a plate of fries in the other. *"I'd like to thank the Academy and Stan's Fries."* Food has always been my buddy, my naughty little secret lover; although I was the only one believing it was a secret, as it was pretty darn obvious to the world judging by the size of me at many moments in my life.

Brantford, Ontario, Canada is my home. Yes that Brantford; home of the Great One and the birthplace of the telephone. Nice Brantford, the Tournament Capital of Ontario and voted Best Blooming City in the world for our municipal floral displays. The Telephone City is home to the Brantford Blast, the Brantford Red Sox, Ball Media, the Wayne Gretzky Sports Centre, Harmony Square, Brant Clown Alley Family Entertainers, Brantford Comedy Fest, Doug (the Great) Hunt -- our 3 time Guinness Record Holder for Stilt Walking and David McKee, our world renowned town crier. Brantford is where you'll find Boomer's Pet Treats, the Brantford Cabaret, Bill's Guitar Skills and Starr Sensations. Brantford is also known for an extremely odd number of Elvis Tribute Artists (ETAs) and showcases, something that I may have directly impacted, and Brantford is home to the Minnery Family. Home is at 117, where I still live in the same house since my birth in February, 1966. Bill and Elsie are my parents. I am the baby sister of John, Anne and Bob. I am the aunt of Alyssa, my brother's daughter. My most worthwhile role is being BJ's mom. Our happy go lucky modest home was lucky enough to have two father figures as our Uncle Joe McGuinness lived with us for over 40 years. He and Pops were a tag team of awesomeness. Mom is the matriarch of 117 in a beacon of music, laughter, comedy, eccentricity and gut-wrenching love. We are cat people. We love the Beatles and Neil Diamond. Our very Catholic home is a photographic shrine to Jesus and Mother Mary, with modest salutes to President Kennedy and Martin Luther King and YES, there are even two floors of Elvis memorabilia.

With the exception of BJ and Alyssa, my family (including Joe) is one full of blue eyes. We all have strawberry blonde hair and are very fair in complexion; however Dad's hair is black, or at least used to be. He's also much tanned. We have all been blessed with killer legs and good teeth, yet we all suffer with bad knees. We have a deep left field belief in the underdog and are all keenly musical. While nobody is a smoker now, our home once was filled with lots of cigarettes, a habit that Mom insisted be broken upon BJ's birth. We were all raised in an Irish Catholic setting where it was the norm to hear comedians on the stereo and Saturday morning records bellowing out Tom Jones and Benny Hill songs. All of us have freckles and are prone to sun burns. We are horrible with vehicles, yet we can all dance very well. Family legacy has an odd President Kennedy connection that lies within a family mystery.

My father, an English Police Bobby Sergeant and my mom, a nurse's aide, emigrated from Liverpool, England with John and Anne in 1953. My sister Anne had been afflicted with the Polio virus and they fled across the pond with a heartfelt desire to find a cure and treatment. Sadly, the Polio had already taken the use of her legs and left her permanently disabled with paralysis.

Mom and Dad set up home in Brantford in the early 50s and a decade later, they welcomed two more children, me and Bob. There are 18 years separating my oldest brother John and me. Basically they had two sets of children. Bob and I became more akin to being the grandchildren. Ironically, John and I were extremely close, while Bob and Anne shared a timeless love bond. Long before I was born, Uncle Joe came to stay with us, supposedly for a week. He never left. Bob and I never knew life without having two male adults in our lives. Uncle Joe was a chubby bloke who loved sweets and potato chips, and found an ally in me as my taste buds were matched equally with his. The whole family would take Bob to hockey and lacrosse; I sat in the stands eating and fantasizing about being a STAR. Huddled in the corner of the hockey rink munching out on chocolate bars, pop and jellied candies, I watched the "movie" of the fantasies I created in my head. I was forever daydreaming about the stage, acting, singing, dancing and marrying whatever heart throb was hot at the moment.

I am quite vertically challenged, standing a diminutive five foot two; one inch taller than my mother. Mom was also known for her gorgeous legs. She had a siren's figure and was a striking woman with her natural red hair and those infamous blue eyes. Dad had black hair, dark complexion and strikingly handsome features. He was always known for his devilish crooked smile. Something else I have inherited along with the same dental palette and chin. Dad was medium average height and build. Mom and Dad were dancers extraordinaire and when they got all decked up to socialize, they resembled Fred Astaire and Ginger Rogers. Mom was blessed with a torch singer's voice and softened a room instantly as she would croon, *"I Really Don't Want to Know."*

My childhood was wonderfully happy, filled with dolls, toys, Hollywood, lots of pink, Elvis, posters of celebrities and one amazing best friend, Joan Harding. Joan lived down the street from me. We became friends when we were 2 years old and to this day, she remains my "bestie." During my childhood, she was with me on an inseparable basis. Joan and I attended different neighborhood schools. I grew up in the Catholic school system at St. Pius School and she attended Prince Charles School. Joan resembled me in many ways: brownish blonde hair (although we both now colour our varying hues of blonde), blue eyes, very white complexion and matching body type. It was that match where our friendship had the greatest bond -- at the fridge. We both loved to eat, as she too had a weight problem. We enjoyed a friendship of many trips to the store for candy and pop, taking walking excursions to the local chip stand or any fast food joint and we were always ordering pizza. Oh, my love affair with pizza. Joan actually reminded me of when we were young teens and we would order TWO pizzas, one for both of us to eat and a small one all for me. We shared a mutual bond of food and loved one another crazily, however not without some drag out cat fights in our younger years. There isn't a piece of my heart that doesn't have her name stamped on it, as she was such an integral part of my childhood. We ventured away from one another in our teens, much to my dismay and sadness, yet always found time to call one another on each other's birthdays and see each other here and there. We found our lives intertwined once again in our forties, when our respective marriages had failed and our parents became elderly. Both of us were once again single and needed to be back at home for various reasons. We share one amazing history together. We have to remain friends, we both know too much!

In a nutshell, I was a fat happy kid who lived in a fantasy world.

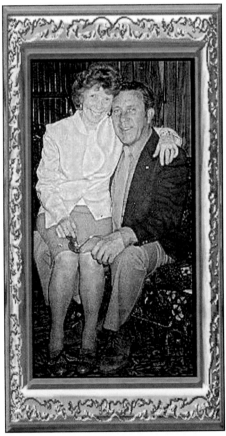

My Parents, Bill & Elsie Minnery
The Wind Beneath My Wings

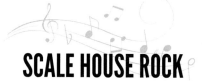

SCALE HOUSE ROCK

In order to answer the frequently asked question about how I changed my life, I need to go back to the beginning, how I ended up a very unhealthy, morbidly obese woman. Have I always been fat? Yes, I have battled the demon for most of my four decades on earth. Apart from a few moments of respite and successful, albeit fleeting, attempts at dieting, I have always lived life large. Obesity does not run in our family, neither on the Minnery side nor the Wilson side. The vast majority of my cousins are medium sized, slender and tall. My mom is quite small, and my grandmother, Marsie Minnery, was only 4'10", so I definitely inherited both of their genes. There's nobody on either side that has severe weight issues, however, my brother John battled weight gain in his adult years after his first marriage fell apart and then had a history of yo-yo dieting. He would always shed it, and then put it back on in direct relation to how his personal life evolved. We share that particular pattern in common.

There's only one reason I was fat: I ate, and I ate a lot. My vices were carbs and salty foods -- cheese flavoured nachos, potato chips, breads, cereals, pasta and what not. While I do enjoy chocolate, it wasn't my vice, although when it was time to have my pity parties, there was always a chocolate bar with me. One main culprit was carbonated pop, mostly in the form of cola. I was also a huge lover of ice cream, although not a gorger; I definitely consumed my fair share of the milky delicacy. I vividly recall when I was younger, sneaking cereal at night and eating bowls of it in the dark secrecy of the bathroom. I have no idea why. I must have known it was wrong, and sneaking it perhaps made it appear to me that nobody was the wiser, telling myself that nobody could hear me. That same sneaky scenario played out down the street, as Joan Harding and I would sneak snacks and binge behind her furnace in the basement. Yes, that is true. There is no denying that I was the pepperoni thief at the Harding homestead as I confiscated umpteen samples out of their fridge. I knew where they were, and I was going in for the kill -- emphasis on the kill. When I was sixteen, I lost a babysitting job completely based upon the fact that I had eaten too many cookies from their house. I also had been sneaking food at several of my other babysitting jobs.

Despite all of this, I wasn't necessarily an inactive child. I played on the odd sports team, and was quite involved with our local St. John's Drum Corps which did lots of marching and walking in parades. I loved playing volleyball and Newcomb ball and thoroughly enjoyed gym class in high school. While I had weight on me and was a husky girl, I had muscle packed legs with the running speed of a horse. I have a trophy collection of red ribbons in the one hundred and two hundred metre races at St. Pius School, and generally advanced to the city track meets where I became known as a running contender. I was quite skilled at baseball as well. I became a respected fielder and home runner. I have never forgotten when two girls on an opposing team lambasted me after sliding into second base; they instantly began hurling spitting laughter towards me while chuckling that my fat tummy was jiggling as I was running. They cut me to the quick causing my eyes to well up as they preyed upon my emotional weakness. While I struck back by hitting a winning grand slam later on during the game, once the season was over, I never went back to play baseball competitively again due to that hurtful moment. Sticks and stones may break my bones, but names will never hurt me. NOT! Hurtful bullying never leaves you. Mind you, years later watching my son BJ excel at baseball and winning MVP during a city wide tournament made me exalt with fist-pumping comeuppance, *"YES! There is a GOD!"*

I had a bicycle and did my fair share of walking, but there wasn't a full activity lifestyle in my daily routines. I also loved to dance and was quite good at it. Of course, there's always the infamous story of when my ballet teacher informed my mother that my "shape" wasn't fit for the delicacies of ballet and that perhaps I should focus more on jazz or tap. I will never forget the pain or the maternal protective love in my mother's eyes as she was lovingly telling me I could no longer take ballet. It is probably one of the most loving and tender moments I have in memory of my mom, second only to her face as she was beside me watching my son being born. Mom tried everything for me to lose weight and slim down. She was always signing me up for any project she could find: laser therapy, hypnosis, ordering weight loss products off the TV. She enrolled me in gym classes at the local Gretzky Centre then dance fit with Carol Kitchen's Dance Centre and eventually the Workout Studio. The Workout Studio was an all-female gym. I loved the fitness classes there and took off with the aerobics craze in the eighties. Aerobics changed how I felt about myself because I could do it well. My ego enhanced and I began feeling confident in myself. Dancing was one of my strongest fortes. Hard core physical fitness became my niche. My body started shifting and I started taking an interest in my health. I became obsessed with aerobics and the love affair of being at the studio which was run by two former models. I relished in the feminine-laced atmosphere; it was intoxicating. Mom's encouragement that I wear one of those "outfits" sparked a fire under my feet as I was decked out in kaleidoscope spandex leotard, body suit, leg warmers and head band. Jane Fonda, *eat your heart out!*

Other than a few teenage crushes and holding hands in the hall way, I never dated in high school. I spent the vast majority of years at North Park Collegiate feeling unwanted, always watching others date and get boyfriends. I was always everybody's buddy; it seemed that everyone preferred my friends. I wasn't a total flop, as I did have a date for the school prom in 1982. My brother Bob even helped accessorize my red taffeta dress and ensured I looked good for my first date. Sad ending: my date stood me up and took someone else. Bob's face as he kept looking at the clock, angrily realizing that my date wasn't coming, is something I will always remember. I'm still waiting for my prom date to pick me up.

Eventually my life took a rather unexpected turn through the arrival of an older teenage boy, *"The Grunt,"* who took my fancy.

Grunt brought about my first kick at the can of a boyfriend and my first heart break. He was the cool guy in the neighbourhood and apparently it wasn't "cool" to date a fat chick. So for six months and all intents and purposes, at least to the outside world, I was just his "friend". (This scenario played out in my life several times over as a heart breaking pattern developed, depleting my self esteem). Grunt's betrayal of me with another girl and his subsequent treatment of me during the Christmas season in 1983 left me shattered. I grieved heavily and the weight piled back on. I secretly abandoned my membership at the Workout Studio; began to hide away from my family and eat. Truth be known, I would walk down the street on the way to the studio, and then veer off to the nearby convenience store to purchase my usual cola, cheese nachos and a chocolate bar. I would then sit on a park bench in Mount Hope Cemetery while gorging everything down. As my tummy grew, it became obvious that I was lying about attending the classes. It was eventually found out and I received quite the verbal lashing from both my mom and sister. The owners of the studio, Patti and Chrissy, encouraged me to return and I promised to recommit.

I returned to the Workout Studio and, while still dealing with the aftermath of my grief over The Grunt, I once again embraced my obsession with aerobics, complete with more outfits and really big hair. I was good at it too and before long I was taking fitness courses to become certified in aerobic dance and fitness instruction. I got hired to teach my own classes, which sent me into a happy tailspin. In fact, teaching anything became my norm. Those fitness classes led me to a long time career in the Brantford area as an aerobics instructor, and a line dancing teacher. I have taught fitness or dancing at a number of local facilities. It is not surprising that life turned that way many years later when the epic weight loss transformation was necessitated. Teaching fitness classes aside, my weight would go up and down like a yoyo, because my life evolved into a constant parade of yoyos.

I developed a knack for getting involved with a bizarre array of wayward waifs. My lost strays would all be the same: lack of jobs, education, driver's licenses, car, rent money, ambition and future. They also had another thing in common: substance abuse problems. I don't drink alcohol, I never have. I also don't smoke and never have, yet for some bizarre, unfathomable reason, my life history has been with clods that drank heavily or were frequent drug users. This parade of strays would suck the money out of my pockets and then cheat on me with their next victim. They were bottom feeders who preyed on good hearted women while also belittling their character. I can't explain why I chose these types of lost sheep. There can be only one feasible explanation; I had such a low opinion of myself that I hooked up with folks that were at the lower end of the food chain because that's where I placed myself. I was never good enough. The humiliation always resulted in more weight gain.

"You get whatever you settle for."

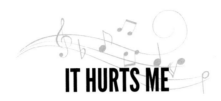

IT HURTS ME

In the summer of 1985, I graduated from Grade 13 at North Park Collegiate and headed off to Mohawk College for the Early Childhood Education (ECE) Program. I had loved and enjoyed high school immensely, surrounded by a wonderful network of friends. I was a happy-go-lucky student and enjoyed sitting on student's council, the camera club and the school newspaper. In my senior years I became a fixture at student assemblies, performing with the vocal ensemble, the school band or solo with simply my voice and my guitar. My academic history had always been that of a decent student, earning myself the Grade 8 Academic Award at St. Pius and the Grade 9 English Award at North Park Collegiate.

College life didn't prove to be a positive experience for me. I enrolled in a course I knew nothing about and instead of going to university to become a teacher, I opted to attend Mohawk College. While this is a fabulous program and institution, my choice in scholastic advancement is a decision I have always regretted. I suppose my regret lies within the decision that I chose to stay close to home because I finally had a real boyfriend and I didn't want to leave him to attend an out-of-town school. Jim and I met during my final year at North Park. In choosing to stay home, I ended up in the wrong program and chose a course that I never truly believed in. Sadly, that choice to attend college instead of university was a silly decision on my part, as my relationship with Jim soon dwindled. Jim was a saint and feasibly the only nice boy I ever knew. I have always wondered if I convinced myself that he was too good for me.

All things considered, I did complete the program and

25

graduated with my ECE diploma. I was twenty two, fresh out of college and took on my first real job working as a School Aide in the Deaf/Blind programme at W. Ross Macdonald School for the Blind, which is commonly known as "the Blind School." The position involved working with the students on three rotating shifts. The evening/night shifts re-introduced horrible eating habits paired with a great deal of inactivity, however, on the positive side, I began making new friends and establishing quality contacts with much of the staff. I eventually took an interest in looking better and I did manage to slim down somewhat.

In the winter of 1989, I was feeling great about myself. I had an awesome job, my first car, new life and new friends. Things were looking up! As my life seemed to go when things went UP – a new guy came into my life. I will refer to him as Lemon. At the beginning of our union, I was a size thirteen. We hit it off quite well at first and seemed to be having a laughter-filled romance, however quite early on I realized that his interest in me began to turn quickly away from being romantic. We spent a year together with him continually shunning me physically. This brought about weight gain and severe feelings of self-loathing. I had a good paying job and very intense feelings for him. It made me easy prey for him to take advantage of my bank account. I desperately needed some form of validation, which allowed him to use me to foot the financial bill for many of his past transgressions, along with numerous gifts and monetary loans. It was a brutal, loveless, one-sided relationship that turned me into a coward and I tried anything to keep my man. That type of treatment and constant rejection continued throughout our entire relationship, as did the one-sided affection. As my fat climb emerged, his resentment towards my increased body weight affected our relationship.

One serious scenario played out at a private gym in Paris, Ontario, when he became physical with me. He was agitated because I wouldn't participate in the workout by using one of the exercise bikes. I preferred to sit on the floor in the gym reading one of the fitness magazines, which irked him. He started yelling at me in the gym, demanding that I get on the exercise bike. I kept reading the magazine; his anger increased, then he started insisting that I get up and weigh-in on a nearby scale. I was extremely embarrassed, felt ashamed and defiantly would not get up. As I was still in the seated position, he grabbed my arms and pulled me across the floor to the front of the scale and ordered, *"Get on that scale! I want to know how much you weigh! How much do you weigh? How much do you weigh?"* Although completely shattered and humiliated, I was brave enough to rebuke his orders to get on that scale. Truth be known, there hasn't been a time since then when I've stepped on a scale without remembering that complete degradation. So, what did I do after he did that to me? What any normal person would do, of course. I co-signed a loan for a new sports car. When I attempted to take the car out once, as it was mine too, he went ballistic and he choked me in the backyard of my home. So, what did I do after he did that to me? What any normal person would do, of course. I asked him to move into an apartment with me. Stupidly, I had stayed with him out of sheer self mortification. To make matters worse, any degree of romance was non-existent as his interest in me was zilch. He avoided me time and time again, resulting in more self indignity, however, the most severe atrocity was about to take place.

We moved in together at the beginning of February, 1990. This coincided with me turning twenty four on February 8. On the evening of my birthday, Lemon and I were sitting on the couch and we began to get cozy. This may seem normal for a young couple, but after a year of dating I was able to count on one hand the number of times we were mutually affectionate. I suppose he decided that because it was my birthday, we would celebrate. He began to kiss me but it became increasingly apparent that he felt awkward. We tried again, but he kept pulling back. I asked him what was wrong. *"I can't do it,"* he shrugged. *"WHAT?"* I cried, *"Why? Why can't you make love to me?"* Then, the man of my life snorted, *"How do you think I feel having to crawl on top of a two hundred pound blimp?"* I was devastated. He disgraced me. When your boyfriend compares you to the Good Year Zeppelin and reveals how repulsed he is by you physically, it impales a wooden stake within your soul. To add insult to injury, in subsequent crying fits, he continually dismissed what he said as being any legitimate reason for my sorrow. He scoffed about how it made me feel. He refused to validate my sadness. He became increasingly distant and moved out, leaving me with a year's lease, rental bills and car payments, resulting in its eventual repossession. His continuous refusal to neither apologize nor accept any amount of blame for what he said broke me into pieces.

I had always been proud of my looks and been comfortable with my very womanly endowments. Lemon convinced me there was something very wrong with me, that I was not good enough, and that I would never measure up. He made me feel that I was not attractive enough to be loved. If I had to choose the defining nucleus of my descent into the obesity Hell that was it. It was the crutch of my rejection, the highest point of my dejection. That defined my entire fat existence and has had the strongest hold of me.

His words resounded in my head and my heart for decades. They were tortuous, made more prolific as they came out the mouth of the man in my life. Due to the utter shame and the humiliation of his rejection, I kept it hidden. I kept that pain secret. In a bizarre twist of fate and a warped sense of reality -- his words DID define me. I grew to become what it was that he called me, a blimp.

"How do you think I feel having to crawl on top of a two hundred pound blimp?"

THIS TIME LORD, YOU GAVE ME A MOUNTAIN

Living through that type of relationship took its toll on my physique and my mind. I became the epitome of self-hate, self-loathing and began eating to dull the pain, and then starving myself into hopes of gaining back his attention. I had to take a stress leave from my job as a Teacher's Aide at the Blind School and became a complete basket case. I went into a rapid downward spiral and the leave of absence was ordered as I dove into a deep, soul-depleting depression. I ended up running off and taking refuge at my sister Anne's home in Ottawa. Anne would always be my Saviour.

It was while on that emotional survival trek in Ottawa that I passed a travel agency and caught glimpse of a holiday magazine with an African lion on the front. One of my life long dreams was and continues to be to travel to Africa. Within the pages of that travel magazine was an ad for the Junior Good Times Club offered through Regent Holidays. Anne and I became quite keen on the fact that the Kid's Club programs were offered at the resorts all over the world. We both felt that time away from Brantford might be best for my recovery. On her suggestion, we wrote to them to see if they were hiring and typed up my resume to accompany the letter. Warp speed ahead -- I had the job 9 days later. Yes, it happened that fast, just like that. I received a call 2 days later, interviewed in Toronto and was hired on the spot. On a whim and a prayer, I quit my job and ran away to the Caribbean to take a job in the Dominican Republic. This is where I began my new life as a Children's Activity Programmer at the Cofressi Beach Resort in Puerto Plata, Dominican Republic.

Fleeing 3,000 miles to the West Indies seemed like a good idea at the time. Arriving in Puerto Plata at the beginning of December, 1990, I was roughly about 180 pounds, having gained some weight during my year with the albatross. Soon though, all of the horror I had been through dissipated upon landing foot on the soil of the Dominican Republic which I called home for two years. I got swept up with the intoxicating music, the Atlantic Ocean, the palm trees, the coconuts, the constant parties at night, the sensual rhythms of the dancing and the allure of the stars floating above the ocean in the night air. I had managed to shed quite a few pounds while I was living in the DR. I was walking and dancing a great deal, living in very poor accommodations and lacking nourishment on a regular basis. This allowed me to shrink down to a size 12. My self-esteem improved along with my confidence.

During my time away, I met Geraldo Sosa Camacho, a 6'1" bronze god of a man. Geraldo and I met at a Club Paradise in February, 1991. The first words out of his brown lips were, *"You beautiful,"* in broken English. Geraldo is a mixture of black and Hispanic. He spoke only Spanish and was a chiseled stallion. I was smitten. I loved the romance of it all. I got totally caught up with the scenario of being in a far away land with a dark lover and living a Harlequin romance novel, so when a dreamy brown guy says those words to a woman who has been rejected repeatedly for being fat, frumpy and ugly, the end result is, of course, to marry him.

On Tuesday, July 16, 1991, in a civil ceremony surrounded by his family, many island friends and the entire activity staff from Cofressi, I said *"I do."* I carelessly married him without thought of anything else other than being married to *someone.* Someone wanted me, finally. Someone found me attractive enough to spend their life with me. In hindsight, I later began to learn that my hapless abandon was merely a band aid solution from within; my subconscious decision to protect myself. I was masking the deep hole in my heart which led me to do what I always joked about doing -- marry the first guy who asked me.

Our wedding was beautiful and so was I. I looked like a fairytale princess. Geraldo said I looked like a white porcelain doll, or as he used to call me, *Muñeca.* On the flip side of the wonderment, there are no words to adequately describe the utter loneliness I felt getting married without my family with me, nor anyone from Brantford. I was by myself on my wedding day, no mother to dress me, no father to walk me down the aisle, no sister to catch the bouquet. The plan was to have a "formal" wedding upon arrival in Canada, once he obtained his immigrant papers. *"Que Pasó?"* I cannot put into context the anxiety I felt sitting in the back of the car while my friend Manuel drove me to the beach side at Costambar. On what should have been the happiest day of my life, it was assuredly my loneliest. The wedding was filled with music and dancing along with the infamous theft of one of the pigs to be roasted, which was carried off by a family of poor Haitian villagers. The next day on our way to Santo Domingo for our Honeymoon, our rental car started on fire and the engine blew up. Omens everywhere!

We found out I was pregnant in November and began preparations for the arrival of our baby that was due the following summer. Three months later, almost tragically, I contracted a tropical disease which developed into acute Cellulitis, resulting in me needing to be hospitalized with growing fears of losing the baby. My body was succumbing to the poison and before I knew it, I was on an emergency flight home with my father at my side leaving my husband on the island for the better part of four months.

William Joseph John (BJ) was born on Saturday, June 27 at 11:35pm at the Brantford General Hospital. His father was off playing baseball in the DR and we couldn't locate him for two days. He did manage to arrive in Canada a few weeks after BJ's birth. From the onset it was obvious that our physical separation had resulted in more than a lack of companionship. I also learned that his Canadian arrival was conditional, due to him testing positive for venereal disease. No doubt this drove a wedge further into the already damaged framework.

My body had grown past two hundred pounds during the pregnancy and I lost faith in myself again with the whirlwind reality that the Dominican romantic flame had dimmed. There were no palm trees, no coconuts, no ocean, no Latin beats into the night; only the reality of two young people suddenly married and raising a child, one of those who did not speak English, was three thousand miles away from home and needed penicillin.

Despite the marital discord, *Our Own Little BJ*, that bouncing baby boy would be the bright light that illuminated our home for the next six months, until darkness was cast by a tragic event that shook 117 down to its very foundation.

On December 12, 1992, my father found his first born, dead in his home. 117 imploded. Our hero was gone. John's death gutted my parents. Poor mom, who had just gotten her right breast removed due to cancer, went into an understandable mental spiral. My father's dark black hair turned grey overnight as he could never get over the sight of his son on the floor, which caused him to drown his sorrows in pints of beer. Our happy go lucky home was demolished. Our once healthy, youthful parents went into immediate decline. Joe tried everything he could to keep the family intact with comedic antics and delving into home repair projects with Dad to keep busy.

John left behind his wife (also named Elsie), his daughter Alyssa and a family overcome with insurmountable grief. Despite the tragic events of his death, he will always remain *"Our John."* His legacy at 117 is one of humour, unparalleled intelligence, knowledge of several languages, infectious laughter, an inability to tell jokes without giggling at the punch line, and a lifetime of memories filled with music and smiles. Yet, there was no escaping the sadness. John's death was akin to shooting off canons through our home and our lives.

Exactly six weeks after John passed away, Geraldo left me and BJ for what we thought was a vacation back home to the DR. On the eve of his return home, I received a phone call from some woman informing me that he was not coming home to Brantford but rather returning with her and moving to Sudbury. Huh? How this all transpired during his vacation, I have no idea, but my understanding is that there was a lot of conspiring going on with him and mutual Dominican friends. I believe that this was planned prior to him leaving. What were his reasons for leaving? According to the mysterious woman, he cited he was not happy in our home because we were crying all the time. What was the truthful reality? He had done his necessary 6 month stay to obtain landed immigrant status and he, like thousands of others similar to him, flew the coop.

My ex-husband (and I use that term loosely) was never an actual *husband*. What I learned was that he merely signed a marriage certificate and did nothing else other than look towards the sky to get on the airplane. Unbeknownst to me, I was married in name only. I wore a wedding dress for a ceremony. Sadly, I was the only person in attendance who was there to get married. There was never an ounce of commitment or any attempt to secure anything past a six month Canadian residency to get landed immigrant status. His only claim is that he provided DNA to help create BJ. I was never "married." I had a legal union with a jackass that used me to get to Canada. I was duped, amidst hundreds of thousands of other women, whom, just like me, believed the lies and the infamous island's story.

I was on the telephone listening to some stranger saying that my husband was not returning. My family was in the kitchen, and upon hearing my one-sided answers, soon realized what was happening. My Dad grabbed the phone out of my hands and gently placed it down on the receiver. He put his hand in my back and eloquently said, *"You stand straight and you never let him see you cry."*

That moment at 117 was the day that our broken hearts began a valiant climb back. We had our hearts pulled through the eye of a needle, first with mom's cancer, then with John's death and suddenly me as a young single mom with a wee baby boy. It turned out to be the best anecdote for 117. That phone call shot adrenaline into the entire family. We'd had enough. We fought back. Mom, Dad, Joe and the Minnery foundation had their new reason for living -- BJ.

"Death leaves a heartache no one can heal, love leaves a memory no one can steal."

33

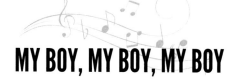

MY BOY, MY BOY, MY BOY

While I had always dreamed of becoming a star and being presented with an Academy Award, God placed life's greatest gift into my arms when he made me a mother. William Joseph John (who we call BJ for Billy Joe), is an extension of my left arm. BJ is my goodness. He is the Earth, fire, water, sky and Moon. He's my breathing. I carried him in my belly for nine months and when that little life sprung out of me, I fell madly in love for the first time in my life. He is the bond between my heart and soul. As I've spent most of my life being stepped on and walked on by countless idiots who stole my faith, it's fascinating how all of that can be instantly evaporated by the eyes of your child staring back at you. BJ's hugs gave me the constant reassurance that to him, I am the world. He made me forget about the loneliness that encompassed my heart.

BJ's arrival came just six months prior to our family being uprooted forever, yet his presence enabled healing and re-established 117 as a happy home. We wrapped ourselves around *"the Beej"* and dedicated our every breath to raising him together in laughter, humour, music and comedic love. He was doted on by everyone and unceremoniously spoiled with never ending attention and inclusion in all activities in town. We enrolled him in everything and learned very quickly that sports and BJ went together like Eddie Van Halen and his guitar, a reference that would surprisingly pop up again when BJ turned 12 years old, as it became excitingly obvious that while he excelled at sports, music was going to be his life's virtuoso.

It is no small wonder that music became BJ's life, as he was surrounded by it from the very start. After all, our entire lives have been enmeshed with music. He was usually with me and my cohorts for most musical adventures while travelling to many destinations and enjoying the wacky life of being the son of "the Elvis Lady." His colourful life was surrounded by men dressed in jumpsuits and women singing doo wop in the basement.

BJ never seemed to be concerned about my weight and I believe it was his inborn protectiveness of his mother that kept his thoughts to himself. While I am positive my growing size had a direct impact on him, it was never verbalized. While he never actually said anything, BJ wasn't immune to being affected by my weight and my developing health issues. On a mom and Scooby (my nickname for him) trip to Niagara Falls, which was supposed to be a three day vacation, our time was cut short, as I had an adverse reaction to an over indulgence of spaghetti and meatballs, then bags of candy and pop which resulted in me having an unfortunate "alien" invasion. I threw up from about 11pm until 5am that night, and had to pack up BJ in the car and drive us both home. I was horizontal in bed for two days. This same scenario played out on other vacations and ruined at least one night while we were on holiday in Disney World where I was again stricken. BJ was only ten years old yet my knight had to walk by himself to the cafeteria to fetch some ginger ale for his mama and stay in the hotel watching TV while I hurled over yet another ivory throne. BJ was very tolerant, yet sadly, I suppose he became used to his mom getting sick. Towards the end of my health bottoming out, there were many nights that found me hurling over my bed into a pot on the floor and keeping the family awake with the loud reefing of my stomach contents.

I can only recall one instance during which there was an exhibition of BJ's abhorrence concerning my weight. BJ and I were going for dinner with a friend of his and her parents. We were taking their SUV and I had to sit in the front. The seat belt would not stretch across me and I could not get it fastened. I laughed it off jokingly, *"That's what you get for putting 15 pounds of mud into a 5 pound bag."* There was an uncomfortable silence in the truck as BJ softly lamented, *"Mommmm."*

Sadly, through all of the musical happiness, I know that the poor dear suffered privately in fear for my life and his, with the reality of his father's absence. Growing up without a father may not have been emotionally easy for *the Beej* but he most assuredly had two amazing role models acting in the father-ship role -- his grandfather and our Uncle Joe. Personally, while I am saddened by his father choosing to be absent, I think BJ got the better end of the deal and lucked out with one hell of a score!

I am eternally grateful that we have had the nurturing and the never-ending support from my parents and Uncle Joe. Despite the obstacles and the roads we could have gone down, we made it. With the single parent scenario, the interracial mumbo jumbo and all of those supposed pitfalls, we made it because of the love that our family has for one another and the magic that is Minnery.

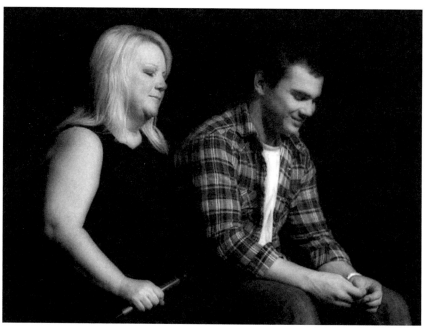

Me and the Beej.
Singing - You Light Up My Life

YOU'LL NEVER WALK ALONE

Once again turning back the clock to the years following John's death, it is no small coincidence that his three siblings turned to music in our individual quests to deal with the grief of losing our brother. One of the greatest gifts that John left behind was his music. John was a wonderfully self-taught piano player. To see this larger-than-life man tinkling on the ivories and singing *Blue Spanish Eyes* was the true essence of a Gentle Giant. As music called us, it was as if John was the orchestra leader from beyond the grave conducting each of us to follow new paths -- all of which were surrounded by melodies. In essence, John sent the harmony.

Bob had always been a music aficionado and had dabbled, rather successfully, in concert promotion. Bob was always a well-liked personality with a vast musical forte. He enjoyed jamming, but the aftermath of John's death would see him delve more into honing his guitar skills and creating his own tunes. Anne, who always loved to sing, began taking singing lessons and writing songs while also joining a choir and a musical cabaret group. Anne later went on to record seven of her own CDs and some of her original work gained radio play in Europe. We always joke, *"She's huge in Holland."*

As for the younger one of the brood, everyone knows I had major aspirations of being a STAR. I loved to sing and did it well. I loved to act, but didn't quite get the whole Strasberg effect. I decided that I would take my grief and turn it into expression through song. With the support of 117, I put together a solo showcase and ventured out into the Brantford spotlight. It dimmed quickly. My first two shows were total bombs, *"epic fail"* as the Beej would say.

Let's just say I neither played to the audience, nor fully investigated my clientele.

For my second attempt, I performed at the Rainforest downtown, a rather uppity and snooty fine dining establishment. Joan Harding was with me and whispered that the man at the bar told the waitress he didn't want to look at me and I was giving him a headache. That same clod went on to inform me, quite rudely, that I reminded him of Rita MacNeil, the Canadian superstar from Cape Breton. He quickly reinforced he was comparing my size and attire to Rita, which cut me down to a new low. Rita was a massively large-sized woman with one of the greatest voices on the planet, yet she was always told that her size and her looks would get in her "weigh." Totally dejected and insulted when a stranger told me the same thing, we packed up the sound system and went home. I believed in my talent and that insult put me into an "I will show HIM mode," and I vowed to get back.

Joan and I joined TOPS (Take Off Pounds Sensibly) together in 1994. I went at it with amazing positive effects and within a year I had shed almost sixty pounds. I can remember BJ's euphoria during my meltdown as I celebrated that my clothes were fitting. He was five years old standing in my room and began jumping on my bed as I tried on different outfits and happily shouted, *"It fits!"* In the end we were both echoing, *"It bloody fits!"* His happy giggles made it one of the lingering close memories within the chambers of my heart. That same year, I also had begun line dancing at Danny's Ho Ho on Friday nights, and attended other classes. I was very keen with line dancing and soon began instructing my own classes and forming a line dancing team called *Dancin' Thunder*. Friday night line dancing is where the Graceliners were born, my female line dancing tribute to ELVIS.

Now, I could go into detail here about my life as a female Elvis Impersonator, my immediate acquisition of the reins of the group and the whirlwind, but that is a whole other book. Suffice to say, this is where my life took on a whole new path and led me to becoming a professional entertainer, special events coordinator and ultimately the Director of the Brantford Elvis Festival. That fifteen year story is fodder for a novel currently in progress. Stay tuned.

A FOOL SUCH AS I

I had a new exhilarating life, I was slim, looking good, and feeling confident in myself. Needless to say, it crept back on rapidly once I went off the rails due to, again, another human being who demoralized my existence.

Enter Effete. I will sum up 'the Effete Effect' with a very real omen that transpired in our home during February of 1998. I had e-mailed an event organizer in Montréal, Québec about having the Graceliners come out to their Elvis Expo, which was on the upcoming weekend. I had sent our bio and was awaiting confirmation that we would be hired and welcome to attend. When the email arrived in my inbox, I went to open the attachment and it shut the computer down immediately. An electrical current went through the house causing lights to flicker. I rebooted the computer and began the entire process again, which shut everything down once more and caused a power surge throughout the house. On my third attempt I was successful in opening the email but the light fixture in my bedroom ceiling was swaying back and forth. At the time, I did not realize that brother John was sending us a warning sign from Heaven, implying impending doom.

There is so much I could say about Effete, and trust me on this, there's a lot that is continually bantered about him by my family, particularly BJ. Effete was a one person wrecking crew. His presence in my life caused me to self-destruct the Graceliners, make bone-headed decisions about my job, turned me into a liar and created disharmony in every corner of my life. When he met me in Québec, I had life in the palm of my hand and was living the dream. When he left there wasn't any semblance of my life intact,

39

and as painful as this is to admit, he had been horrifically unkind to BJ, causing my baby boy to be in fear around him.

Losing the Graceliners and all cohesiveness of my life caused me to mentally implode and eventually my body began to explode. However, something good came out of all of that. I vowed that Effete would be my last. I was never again going to allow anyone to treat me like a doormat. I was fed up with maxing out my bank account for men who treated me as if I was gum at the bottom of their shoes. I was slamming the door and locking the key. I promised myself that I would remain single until such a time when God finally kicked the Devil to the curb and brought somebody in my path worthy of my heart.

Then the eating took on a dismal life of its own.

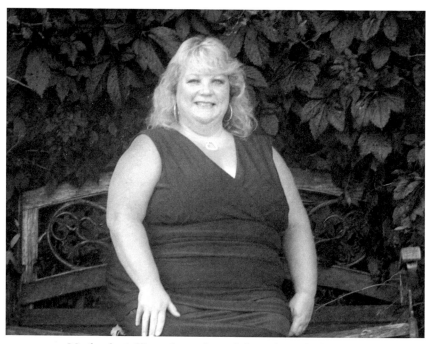

My body telling the tales of decades of abuse...

WALK A MILE IN MY SHOES

In 2000, we lost Uncle Joe to stomach and liver cancer, another event which shook 117 to its very foundation. His death came as such a shock to all of us as it happened so quickly. We found out he had cancer in July and he was gone by December. Watching one of the world's gentlest men suffer the way he did was very traumatic and painful. Joe was so kind, full of humour and pure goodness. People as remarkable as Joe, should never have to die like that. Joe's death was intricately difficult on all of us but *'the Beej'* took it especially hard. Joe and BJ were best buddies and were always together. His death left a void in 117 but his life left a legacy that will always be cherished. Ironically, one of the last conversations I had with Joe was him begging me to get healthy and to promise him that I would not to allow BJ to do what he and I had done to our own bodies.

While still recovering from Hurricane Effete, I did manage to start a new singing group called *Memphis Motion,* a salute to Elvis and the '50s and '60s. Having gained a great deal of popularity with the Graceliners and becoming a regular featured entertainer here in town, I was able to quickly market MM as we began to dominate the performers' line-up in Brantford and Ontario. What an eclectic array of singers and performers we had -- which I will reserve for the *next* book.

I also began teaching Vocal Music at the Ontario Conservatory of Music, forming my own youth group, Starr Sensations. Before I knew it, my young protégés were scooping up singing awards and my career as a music educator took off on its own orchestrated journey. Eventually I started working for myself and opened up my

41

own home based business -- the Starr Sensations Vocal Studio. I geared my professional life towards leading young children to music.

The *Brantford Elvis Festival* opened up to rave reviews in 2000 and we welcomed 8 more festivals to town, with a tourism award for Best Festival and Event in 2004 and I also won for Best Tourism Builder. I have also been honoured with being a two-time finalist for the Brantford Expositor's Citizen of the Year and receiving countless accolades and civic awards from the municipality.

To the outside world, I had it all. My professional life was seemingly successful; we were touring, garnering fans from all over Canada and the United States and we welcomed an exhaustive performance schedule. My role in MM was as the director and lead singer. I played the big lady with the big voice and infectious flirty persona. Everyone raved about my Energizer Bunny stage antics and how happy go lucky I appeared.

On stage I was the Sgt. Major in control. The reality was that as my professional life soared, my personal life tanked. I was a very public figure with a very "public figure." I wore a mask of success but behind the veil was another story that was hidden from everyone. It is behind a person's eyes where the truth lies - and mine was a tale that nobody knew.

Being a large-sized woman in the entertainment field is not easy. Being a big woman alongside other big women and expanding waist bands from our Elvis Tribute Artists (ETAs) brought about some misfortune. While our dream team harmonized in excellence, we had some rather disturbing occurrences that boomeranged across all of us. We were all hurt by the onslaught of nastiness. However, as the director I had to deal with them head on. Perhaps all of this caused me to take bigger hits due to the fact I had never properly dealt with my own heaping issues.

While performing at Carmen's Banquet Centre during the Fireman's Ball, a young blonde gal began laughing hysterically at me in my mini-skirt and high heel boots only to lose it more upon seeing the rest of us appear. That was nothing compared to the soul-wrenching evening in Mitchell, Ontario at the Nurse's convention. An extremely rude petite brunette burst out shouting,

"Are you ALL fat? Are we going to have to look at your fat all night?" Having to suck up fat comments from audience members, albeit fleeting, plays havoc on your self esteem. I loved entertaining and we were great, yet I wasn't mentally prepared for the backlash of being obese and trying to entertain crowds.

We continued to garner awards and gain more shows despite the fact that an e-mail campaign began in my inbox from an anonymous naysayer who wrote that he thought we "should find other careers where we could be heard and not seen." He continued by saying that Memphis Motion was nothing more than laughing stocks, our appearances were a joke and that while we did have some talent, we should do everyone's eyes a favour because nobody wanted to see our fat jiggling. We did end up identifying the hateful individual, but by then, the damage had already been done.

People never truly realize that what they say can break your heart. In 2002, while performing at the Casino Windsor, I had just brought down the proverbial house with a full capacity standing ovation after my rocking rendition of Janis Joplin's *Me and Bobby McGee*. At the end of the show, two middle-aged women came up to me, seemingly ready to raise kudos about my performance, as I was being congratulated by many. The silver-haired woman calmly said, *"You should try doing Mama Cass; you have the look."* I don't know who wanted to crawl under the rug more, me or my singing partner standing next to me who tried in earnest to explain that the woman had said that because Cass Elliott was an incredible vocalist. NO, she did not. Just like the man who had insulted me at the Rainforest, once again, it was about my size.

There are some things that are hard to admit, but this story is about putting it all out there, in hopes of waking people up. I'm trying to hit home with others using the same boat in which I used to sink. There's a whole lot of fat-related stress mess to which persons who are overweight must own up. While my life in the spotlight has been all sequins, big hair, vanilla perfume, glamour and glitz, being fat is NOT glamorous.

While it's never been spoken about, as I morphed, it became more difficult to maintain adequate daily hygienic routines, particularly, if I was in another bathroom with a toilet other than my own. Due to my growing rear end and the abnormality of my tummy hang, being able to effectively wipe myself became a chore. I vividly recall having to undress myself in the bathroom at Union Station and needing to cock my leg up on the toilet paper dispenser to be able to maneuver myself into a position to reach my behind. I failed and had to return back to a vehicle full of friends, which resulted in a very uncomfortable ride home. That scenario played out time and time again. I never listened.

One of the worst moments that brought me to tears happened in my sanctuary at App's Mill Nature Centre in Paris, ON. App's Mill is my nirvana. It is a place where I found sanity and serenity and have cried rivers of tears and have also done a great deal of eating. I love the outdoors and trails near water are continually tranquilizing to me. It was summer time; I was in shorts. As I was walking along the trails, I had to climb up an embankment which caused me to climb even more quickly and I heard this "swishing" sound. I didn't know what it was. About five minutes later, I climbed down another embankment, causing me to somewhat run near the end. I heard the "swishing" sound again. The water must have been drowning out the sound before. Now I was a good distance away and in a clearing. I could hear it on a regular basis, especially as my left leg was moving forward. I painfully shrieked as I found out that the sound was my fat swishing against my thighs and my belly was flopping against my skin making the now identified horrific sound. I sunk onto a log and cried. I vowed to get better. I never listened.

Of course there's always the overlooks: When you get passed over by a suitor who slams you with the infamous, *"You're pretty; you should lose some weight."* Or the all too familiar, *"You're not quite what we're looking for,"* said the captain of the high school cheerleading squad laughing at you, despite having successfully executed every routine with finesse, including the splits and the cartwheel. Also, let's not forget the insensitive teenage boy who blurted out at Prince Charles Park, *"I'd date her if she didn't have all that fat hanging out below her shirt."*

None of the overlooks amounted to the bittersweet disappointment of one of my life's most embarrassing letdowns.

While on the road with Memphis Motion in 2008 for our Nashville Tour, I came down with a flare up of the mysterious "alien" brought on by a barrage of candy and crap purchased at a truck stop, which spawned an attack 3 hours later. Memphis Motion was scheduled to appear at the Gaylord Opryland Hotel, which I had to cancel, as I was upchucking in the hotel room. We took fifty people to Nashville with us to see us perform; I was puking into a waste basket while my two team members were left on their own for what should have been our greatest performance and chance at the "big time." What made matters worse, is that the following night, I was also far too sick to accompany Memphis Motion to perform with the live band at the Nashville Nightlife Dinner Theatre. BJ is a brutally honest chap and there has been several times in our lives when he's given me the "what for" gears while maintaining his overwhelming mama's boy smile. BJ sure did give me a stern talking to that evening, followed by a tearful plea for me to *"get some help"* from my Elvis Tribute Artist friends Bob and Marilyn Hajas. I boarded that bus back home in disgust with myself, and a head hung low in self pity and self absorption. Upon returning home, it was identified that the "alien" I had been suffering from for years was developing pancreatitis. My family doctor warned me that I had an impending stroke coming within a year if not sooner. I vowed to get better. I never listened.

The attacks had become so severe that I began missing shows due to my increased 'alien' invasions. I also ended up being rushed to Emergency three times. The last time I was there was the most pathetic. I had to have two extra blood tests because the first blood test was unable to be accurately processed. The reason: the blood vial was filled with FAT on the top half of the vial and the technicians could not properly analyze my blood. The on-call doctor, again, told me that my readings were off the charts and that she was horrifically worried that she would see me back up there in the near future but it wouldn't be in E.R, it would be in the morgue. I vowed to get better. I never listened.

The attacks began sparingly for a few years but they gradually began to increase in frequency and longevity. As already stated, BJ became accustomed to me falling prey to the "alien" on every vacation, after I had gone off the rails with my eating, and seemingly being very careless in the sun and eventually ending up horizontal and green. I vowed to get better. I never listened.

The attacks weren't the only aspect of my health that left me suffering. My blood pressure began to escalate, especially under the hot spotlights of the stage. I am quite active when I perform, and my weight never slowed me down in that matter. My agility however, was becoming more laboured and my face was turning purple, which caused audience members to squirm. A husband and wife team revealed that they would literally sit and wait for me to collapse. Out of fear that I was going to stroke out, one of them wouldn't leave to go to the bathroom when I was on stage. I vowed to get better. I never listened.

While dancing and rehearsing for a play in Delhi in 2009, I suffered a mild cardio episode, which prevented me from carrying on and left me breathless for hours. I was very scared. I vowed to get better. I never listened.

While dancing in a similar show, on the same stage the following year, I had a fall 10 minutes before curtain, causing me to land on both of my knees and end up horizontal on the ground. I was in a Humpty Dumpty state. I could not get myself up as I rocked back and forth unable to do anything except roll to and fro. That same evening, my jeans split during one of the numbers. Embarrassingly, the jeans had an elastic waist-band. I vowed to get better. I never listened.

My good friend Ty Humpartzoomian had quite the heart to heart talk with me about my weight gain and how MY weight was affecting ALL aspects of my life. I think because the talk came from a man and someone I trust and am very fond of, it hit home. His words were so gentle and caring as he rather angrily told me, *"Joanie, you're poisoning your body. I'm getting really pissed off with you. It's making me madder and sadder every time I see you, because you are continuing to grow."* Although the words caused my eyes to swell up, I knew they were said out of respect for me as a person and also out of concern. His words truly echoed loudly and reverberated. I vowed to get better. I tried to listen.

G.I. TRACT BLUES

I ate in excess because I was living a happy life on stage while the reality was that off stage, I hated myself. I hated my life and having two personas began tearing me apart.

Being fat was the only me I knew. I got used to it and succumbed to being an obese person. Complacency included avoiding my naked body in the mirror and covering it up with dark clothing. To combat my body, I dyed my hair platinum and styled my mane like Farrah Fawcett. I would put on dazzling make-up to create stand out blue eyes and glossy lips. All I had was my face and my golden locks. When the triple chin crept up on me, I accentuated my figure with push up bras to reveal my very ample cleavage and I doused myself with glitter. Two thirds of me was a disaster but the upper third looked like a Las Vegas showgirl.

There is no question I was a food addict. I ate a *lot* and most of what I consumed was junk and unhealthy fast food. The biggest binges generally occurred in the evening or at night. I accepted and lived with my body. Due to not having "love," I learned to love food and obviously didn't love myself enough to comprehend and conceptualize that what I was eating, not to mention the amount, was slowly killing me.

Prior to my weight loss journey, I rarely ate breakfast. I would start eating at noon and didn't stop until midnight. I snacked and nibbled and gorged and my body was a direct reflection of that. I was known as the person who sat down at the dinner table, rarely lifted my head up from my plate, inhaled my food, and then got up and walked to the counter to make toast. There was no denying the reason I was fat; it was because I ATE. I was one hell of an eater!

As I grew out, I indulged in secret (or so I thought) late night trips to the fast food restaurant or the pizza parlour just up the street from my house. I would sneak outside into my car, not closing the door in fear of someone hearing the door shut, I would hold it with my left hand, not turning on the lights but then stupidly putting the key in the ignition and starting the engine. The irony of that now makes me giggle. I wasn't fooling anyone. Those late night trips would always lead to me either having a two slice box of pizza and a coke or happily venturing off to King George Road for my usual fast food devouring of a fish fillet, fries and a cola or a milk shake. These treats were furiously shoved down my gullet and gobbled up within 5 minutes; basically it was insert food and swallow.

In 2009 my life and health had plummeted and all hope within me began to dwindle. Through years of neglect, my health had been growing intensely worse, my vision became affected and my once controllable tummy disturbances were now increasing with intensity and frequency. I couldn't walk for long periods of time, nor climb stairs without having great difficulty breathing. I had spent almost ten years suffering from staggering pancreas, gall bladder and liver issues. A new crop of serious issues developed with acute vertigo and vision ailments. My face was always red with high blood pressure and my nights were spent choking from severe gastroesophageal reflux disease which is known as GERD (white foam coming up through throat and out of the nostrils). I was also suffering from overwhelming mental depletion. I probably was crying out inside and hoping for some form of recognition from secretive sources that I was suffering and in need of medical assistance so that I could have the attention I was craving. *"OVER HERE...look at me dying over here. Maybe NOW they will notice."* It never worked. It only made it worse.

I spent twenty years topping the scales at well over 200 pounds, which eventually morphed to a staggering scale reading as I had eaten myself up to almost 300 pounds. I was losing my will to live. I had lost every life desire and had given up on myself. My health was staggering out of control; every organ, every fibre of me was aching and my body was beginning to react and back up. I knew that my body was about to quit.

As a lifetime of hurt was sitting on my shoulders, I got used to it and I became accustomed to being hurt and abusing myself. It was the norm. I ate to kill the pain. I ate out of loneliness, frustration, anxiety, stress and the overwhelming feeling of abandonment. My early forties left me shaken up and horribly wounded. I felt like I did not matter and ended up treating myself as such.

I teach musical theatre and even that had become a chore and a source of stress. As a single mom, BJ had resigned himself to the fact that he was going to live his adult life without his mom. Doctor's appointments were in abundance as well as testing and examinations by medical specialists. We had been told by many health professionals that I was a walking ticking time bomb and nothing was hitting home, not even the completely demoralizing truth that my ability to maintain regular daily hygiene was being compromised by my size and my obvious declining health.

I could not see a way out of the Hell I was living. My overwhelmingly low self-esteem was being compounded by self-defeating emotions, which led to a total loss of control over decision-making related to my career and matters of the heart. It was a horrific year for me, feasibly the lowest ebb of my whole life. Quite honestly, there was a point in December 2009 when I just wanted to find a clearing somewhere and lie down.

All of this was having a runaway train effect on my psyche. My heart had been pulled through the eye of a needle. My life was beginning to unravel, as I was making alarming and out of character choices surrounding my professional and personal life. These included abandoning the Starr Sensations choir, taking a leave of absence from teaching and diminishing my roster.

Finally, the most critical of decisions came with the obvious need to end Memphis Motion. As the director and lead singer of the group, my role was as captain. All bookings, all business dealings, negotiations, music collaboration, planning and all functions belonged to me. While we had a tremendous support team of volunteers at shows, and extremely dedicated cast mates, my duties weren't just as a singer, they were as the main controller. That was also the case when on stage. I was a clown, almost behaving as a

Bette Midler-type of on stage personality: manic, loud, boisterous, outrageous, silly and flirty. It was my responsibility to be the person to get the crowd going and do anything for a laugh. Some of my best acting roles were within those shows. The character on stage was never the real person off stage. It caused confusion as my quietness and aloofness off stage was misconstrued as a coldness or inapproachability. The reality is that it became exhausting to carry that falsehood onto the stage and also carry the show when my true reality was the direct opposite. A person can only hide the truth for so long. It caught up with me and our shows began to suffer, as did my commitment to the direction.

Memphis Motion was not a happy team any longer. Nobody is to blame. Nobody was right, nobody was wrong. We were together for thirteen years with a revolving door of cast mates. Our touring schedule and lackluster performances became mundane resulting in everyone feeling burned out, including our audiences. This caused anxiety of astronomical proportions. I agonized and ate myself into a deeper depression. I was under intense emotional stress in making that decision. In retrospect, as I look back, the more irrational behaviour was in holding onto MM for as long as I did; it should have been disbanded two years earlier. I was trying in vain to hold on to it like a sort of life preserver, as I was ebbing. As cliché as it was -- I was caught in a trap and I had to get out.

Truth be known -- I had given up. I was so desperately reaching for help but nobody was listening mainly due to the fact that I was too embarrassed to admit it.

There is no doubt that I have been blessed with a rather staggering successful professional life, yet my personal struggles with depression and food dependency shattered my heart for decades. The outside world knew me as glamour and glitz while I was really suffering in silence and loneliness. I could no longer separate my two worlds, as my body started to give out and my mental depletion caught up with me.

I lost all confidence in myself as a musician and as teacher, an event promoter and in everything, Joan. My decreasing lack of self respect led me to make uncharacteristic choices which caused a rippling avalanche.

There are some things better left unsaid. Some hurts go too deep. Suffice to say, a phantom appeared as I veered towards the point of no return. I felt myself evaporating into demonic quick sand. It all came crashing down around me. I had hit rock bottom. And then the dam burst; literally, it busted.

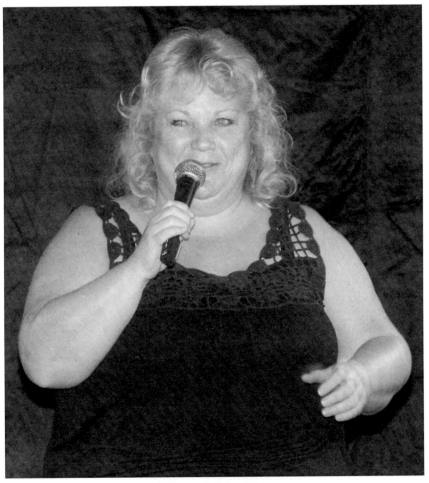

August 27th, 2010
The day the journey began..

ALL SHOOK UP – THE A-HA MOMENT

Everyone has their wake up call, their "A-HA" moment. Their fed up, shake up and get an intervention moment. Mine occurred in August of 2010, when I was undergoing a "routine" Meniere's syndrome test at a medical clinic in Hamilton, Ontario, another test to find out the root of a problem we all knew. FAT was killing me. My best friend FOOD was causing a domino effect -- suicide through suicide chicken wings. As excruciating and invasive as the test was, I was blasé about the whole thing, until my world was tipped on my axis and my insides came out. I had an adverse reaction to the test and spewed my breakfast all over myself, the nurse and the walls of the clinic. Upon sitting up, I wet my pants and before I could get off of the examining table, my bowels opened up. If I had to compare the humiliation of that feeling to anything, I felt like Carrie from the Sissy Spacek horror film of the same name, when she is covered in pig's blood. I sat there in a freaked out state, put my head down and cried, *"I didn't sign up for THIS."* There is no greater realization of self-loathing than to be faced with the reality that you are forty minutes from home, have no change of clothes, are by yourself in another city and have to drive yourself down a highway with poop and pee in your pants, and vomit in your hair.

I sped to the bathroom of the medical clinic and saw the aftermath of my soiled black shorts (I was dressed as if I was in mourning) and pushed my bloated feet into my flip flops. Frantically trying to clean myself up in unfathomable embarrassment, I rushed out of the clinic and made a bee line to our burgundy van which now screamed "sanctuary." With fingers trembling, a foggy head and a tummy fighting back more bile upchucking; I called home but didn't get any answer. I texted BJ to call me on the cell phone right away.

It was August on a hot afternoon so I kept the windows open. I tried to forget the stench. I tried to forget that I could feel the fecal matter in my panties and see the remnants of it on my legs. I pushed away the smell of the urine and the uncomfortable reality that I was sitting in my own filth. As much as I tried to avoid the mirror – I saw me. I saw the green sea-sick look on my pudgy ashen face. I saw the three chins. I saw the eyes that were sunken and almost invisible in a swollen face. I could see the stained tracks of tears cemented into my cheeks from months of emotional turmoil. Looking back at me I saw someone much older than my 44 years. I wept. I felt horrifically sorry for myself. What I did *not* feel was responsible. What I felt was angry. I was angry at the nurse for putting me through that test. I was angry at my doctor for sending me to have the tests. I was angry at everyone who made me eat. I was angry at the throngs of friends who had betrayed me. I was angry at the men who had used me and who treated me with disregard. I was angry at the test. I was angry...

Then the phone rang. BJ was on the other end. I pulled over on Highway 403 at the Copetown exit and harshly ordered, *"Beej run me a bath I've had an accident."* *"What do you mean you've had an accident?"* he queried. *"Beej, I've had an accident, please run me a bath."* *"I don't understand Mom, a car accident?"* Frustrated I roared down the phone, *"NO!!! I've crapped myself, run me a bath."* I could hear his voice trailing off as I hung up.

What I failed to realize and rationalize is that the person I was most angered with was ME. I had done this to myself. My body was finally done; it had given up. The pancreas had had enough. It was over, it was done. I was done, we were done. My beaten body had backed up and had come through every opening it could find. Sadly, the most obvious opening was the window to my soul. My once breath-taking blue eyes were now grey. The cute face I had possessed was wrinkled with chubby fat deposits and years of self abuse. I looked dishevelled. I wore the long results of apathy.

I cried again. I lamented what was happening. The smell

became intrusive. I could not escape from it. I began to drive faster, as if going quickly would allow me to be successful in fleeing from the pungent whiffs of my own internal sewage. I sunk into my seat and into the waste within my underwear and the hardening of feces that had dripped and coagulated on my legs. As I pulled off the highway and turned onto Morton Avenue, all I could think of was the bath. I could wipe this all away. I could strip off and clean myself up and go to bed. I was ready to heave again and knew I was going to have a few more hours of illness and would probably end up horizontally bed ridden.

Gunning the engine through the lights at West Street and into our neighbourhood, I could see BJ in the distance standing in the driveway. He was waiting for me. *"I'll just rush past him, he won't notice anything,"* I thought to myself. *"I've got this, just act like nothing is wrong."*

Bitter reality hit me when I pulled into my driveway. BJ's face turned sour. *"Mom, I could smell you coming up the street, what the hell happened to you?"* He stared at me in disgust and disbelief. As I timidly got out of the van, my predicament caused a facial reaction from him that I NEVER want to see again. He immediately saw the pasty look of ailment on my face, the pee stained shorts -- and then he saw the feces. I was sheepishly moving into the house as his knees buckled at the sight of his mother with poop running down her leg. *"Mom...Mom, what the—you-you-you're dying!"* His brown eyes welled up with tears. I hung my head in shame. *"I know,"* I cowered, hurrying into the house, BJ in pursuit sputtering questions about how I ended up in that state. I couldn't speak out of humiliation and anguish. I was immobilized. Then, out of the mouth of my baby, came the words that changed my life, now and forever. He grabbed hold of both of my elbows, eyes dripping with moisture. With loving venom seeping from his tongue, he feverishly snarled into my face, ***"STOP KILLING MY MOM. When are YOU going to STOP mom? YOU are killing my MOM! STOP KILLING MY MOM!!!"***

Seeing BJ's eyes and his desperate attempt to shake me up, I came face to the face with the deep realization that the person I was hurting MORE than myself was my son. He was in a fearfully panicked state about losing his mom. His horror combined with the heartfelt pleas during his voluminous tirade snapped me into focus. I had done this to myself. I was responsible for the poison. I WAS killing his mom. My most important person in the entire universe was going to lose HIS most important person and it became up to ME to prevent that from happening. I was staring eye to eye into his future without me. At THAT moment, everything for me changed.

Forty four years of crap had piled up. There's no denying it. I had been crapping on myself for years as I allowed and invited the crap in. It was no wonder that on the day of the 'A-HA' moment the organ that gave way was my bowels. As I ended up literally crapping on myself, I had a painful epiphany. *"ENOUGH IS ENOUGH."* I knew better. I was educated, bright, articulate and smart. I knew better. It was all being reflected upon my body and my skin. Time for me was running out. I knew it was time to grow some balls, take back my life and gain control.

My life was a book in which I no longer wished to be the main character. I had a simple choice to make, to write a sob story or a success story. In order for me to pen that Pulitzer, I had to first get out of my own way! It was time for me to change my story, not just the next chapter, but compose an entirely new book.

It is vitally important to implore upon my readers and everyone who knows about my story that my "A-HA" moment did not occur in the medical clinic. It did not occur on the ride home or when my bowels opened upon me. It didn't even occur pulling into my driveway. I was still in denial. It was the look on my son's face and his words of fierce compassion as if he would die himself if he lost me. BJ reached into the depths of his soul bypassing his heart and with the intensity of the greatest guitar solo; he ERUPTED at his mom in a last stitch attempt to intervene. When he cried to me, *"STOP KILLING MY MOM,"* he wasn't yelling at me, he was reaching inside of me to pull the REAL me out. I had become a morphed up version of a shell of who I used to be. I was merely an encasement of the Joan Minnery that used to exist. His pleas were as if he was hollering down a 100 foot man hole painfully calling to me to ask if I was still alive; hoping with every fibre that I answered.

I wasn't just killing his mom. Through my abuse of me, and the subsequent mental anguish and total loss of anything familiar to Joan, his mom was also threatening to kill him. Not in body, but in spirit and in emotional distress. On that hot August afternoon in 2010, within the confines of our driveway at 117, my young 18 year old son grew into a man and my saviour. As I had given him life, he was now valiantly saving mine.

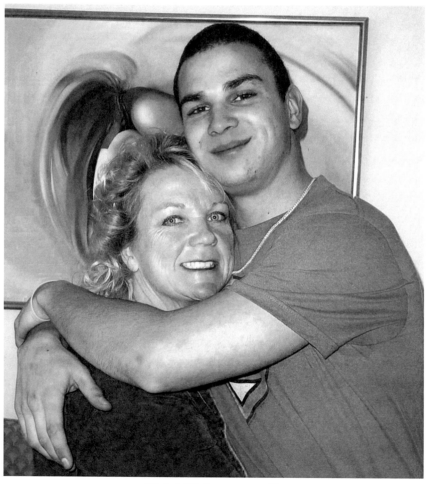

He's MY Superman!!!

FIT

Listen, Lord Jesus let my fears be few.
Walk one step before me, I will follow you.

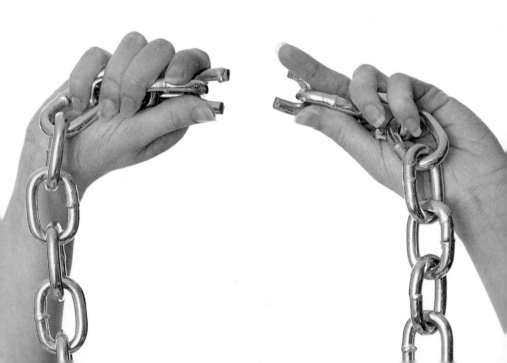

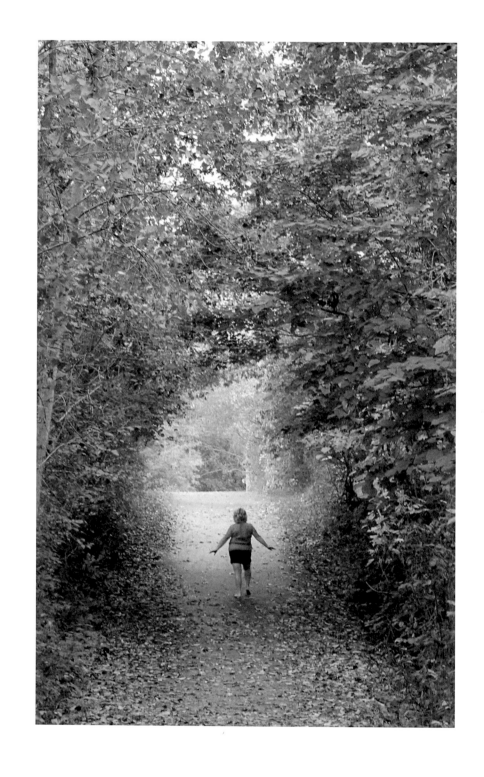

THE COMEBACK SPECIAL

With the painful realization that I was standing in front of my son and my parents, with feces dripping down my leg, the voice I had been longing to hear finally broke through and emerged following a number of sad sighs then acceptance. I suddenly found myself within the long-awaited "A-HA" moment.

My melancholy shoulder hunch morphed into an eerie head raise that was joined by a powerful phoenix, whose rising voice said words that resonated within me. A haunting phrase sprung up from the very depths of my mind and the core existence of Joan. I uncrossed my arms in front of me and whispered these words into the palm of my left hand which was now at my mouth. My lips were moving feverishly as the words came out. I said the phrase, several times over again. A mantra for my journey was born, which continues to be a constant source of motivation. These words have been the fire within my soul, the burning ember that nobody can extinguish which grows stronger with every pound lost and every smile gained. No fanfare, no glaring trumpets, nobody heard them except for the three most important people who finally needed to - me, myself and I. What were these words? *"They've seen you at your worst; let them see you at your best."* As I rose from the ashes I enacted a plan.

When one goes off in search of themselves, it is imperative and necessary to locate the moment when they first lost themselves. I'm not certain this book ever truly indentifies that moment, but it definitely outlines the long journey and a series of unfortunate events that eventually led to the definitive moment where I not only had lost myself, but also lost my mind, my spirit, my music and ultimately hit rock bottom. Once I had hit it, I had to find my way home. I had to be HONEST with myself. I had to find out the true reason I was eating, going deep within myself through meditation, prayer and cathartic stimulation. The truth was easy to spot. I was morbidly obese, looking the absolute worst I have ever looked and dangerously unhealthy. I had endured a procedure that completely annihilated me and was undergoing tests upon tests in one medical facility after another. My tummy was spewing a lifetime of poison back up on a daily basis. There was clearly only one way to stop the cancerous bulldozer of death and that was to stop the insanity. My life was filled with too much negativity and depression and I had to turn it around. I was fed up with being sick, tired of being used and I became cynical about my own self-worth.

I was fat because I ate. I was morbidly obese because I ate a *lot*. There is no denying the reasons for me being overweight. It was because I gave up on me. As folks or situations hurt me, I took out all aggression on myself. I suppose I can blame my weight gain on years of freaking imbeciles invading my heart, but the reality was such that I couldn't keep blaming them. I chose to eat. I, not anybody else, did it to myself. I think what I was doing was creating my own coat of armour -- the fat was there as a way of keeping others out. I created a shield around me that nobody could penetrate and that was my armour, my armour of fat. If I looked *that* way, nobody could hurt me.

There's no denying I lead a hectically busy life, yet the life I was living was the life of a thin person and to be honest, I could no longer sustain my life supported by the frame on which I stood. Something had to give before my pancreas gave out. At the time, I truly had no idea where I was headed. I just knew that the path I was on was leading to broken promises and dreams; certain death, quite literally. It was time to reverse years of damage I had done to my body. I decided to raise the standards for myself and live differently. It was time to lick my wounds, repair the injuries and improve my whole system.

I made a commitment to myself and to everyone that is important to me, that it was time to get really serious about my future. I was fed up living a lonely life and I was ready to get healthy. I knew that immediate changes were needed. On Friday, August 27, 2010, while standing in the Grand Ballroom of the Best Western during the *Rock of Ages* Festival in Brantford, I started on a health and wellness journey. I began *WALKING MY WAY BACK TO ME*.

I was well known for not eating during events. I would refrain from ingestion due to severe diarrhea, a result of stress and nervousness. I could not eat anything. No matter what major multi-day event I was producing, it was a tradition for me not to eat during those times and this made way for the plan to be welcomed. It was controversial. It was radical, but it also enabled me to purge, cleanse and detoxify. My healthy eating plan began the morning after the *Rock of Ages* festival was complete and it was planned that way on purpose. I had also announced I was ceasing the festival. I knew I was walking away. I had made that life-altering decision weeks before and I knew that I was shutting it all down. All of the Elvis shows, all of the tribute contests -- done! Clean slate, clean house, everything shut down. A new life meant just that -- a *NEW* life!

After having put together countless award-winning productions, always being in charge, always being the producer, I was now the entire production crew in putting together the greatest return since Elvis appeared in his leathers in the infamous '68 comeback special. I was 44 years old starring in MY own version -- The "44" comeback special.

"The soul always knows what to do to heal itself, the challenge is to silence the mind." – Caroline Myss

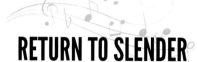

RETURN TO SLENDER

"Joan how did you lose all that weight?" "What's your secret?" "What diet are you on?" "What did you do to lose that much?"

My friends, I wish I could tell you about a magic pill that you take before bed, resulting in a slimmer figure by dawn or magic beans that you ingest that allow you to eat everything in sight and never gain an ounce. Wouldn't it be awesome if doctors were able to bottle the metabolism of skinny people and cure us folks who gain weight simply by walking past a hot dog cart? Unfortunately, that's not reality. The bitter truth is that if you're vastly overweight, it's going to take time and it's going to take one heck of a commitment to yourself to see it through to the finish line.

I don't have any secret remedy. As far as I know, there isn't one. The only working remedy out there that is 100% fool proof is back-to-basics, no-nonsense healthy eating and exercise. No gimmicks, no fancy pills, no medical intervention in the way of clinical procedures or weight loss centres. No shakes, no products, no fancy programs, no quick-fix remedies, no two thousand dollars a year memberships -- just plain old-fashioned common sense dieting combined with movement. I have done this 100% on my own through the help of my weight loss guru -- the local grocer. The first order of business was my diet. I'm not going to lie; restricting my food intake required a lot of willpower. Let's be honest, I was fat my entire life. I knew what I had to do and how to do it; anyone who is overweight knows what to do. Simple math, do the opposite of what you are presently doing. I'm willing to bet every dollar I've spent on cola, that almost every fat person knows exactly how to lose weight. If we put it on, we know how to take it off. This is not rocket science; it's all about re-educating yourself, and using what you already know. Successful weight loss and dieting equals common sense eating.

So, how did I lose all that weight? My changes were as follows:

- Start every day with breakfast. Never skip breakfast

- Eat Breakfast. Eat A Big Lunch. Eat A Small Dinner

- Eliminate eating past 8pm

- Ensure that I have 3 meals, including protein

- Up protein - If it runs, swims or flies -- EAT IT!

- Fish/seafood, chicken/turkey, beef and pork, in that order

- Lower carbs

- No indulging in chocolates, cookies, chips or any of the good stuff

- Stop drinking all pop. That eventually included diet too!

- We need carbs and taking them out of any person's diet is ridiculous. It's the cause of the failure of so many diets. I have them with limits and eat the carbs in the morning and the early part of the afternoon. They are needed for energy later so they store up and release over time.

- Cease ALL visits to the drive-thru at fast food chains, unless choosing healthy alternatives. No greasy drive thru hamburgers or fish filets. Eliminate all deep-fried foods including southern chicken. ALL GONE!

- Eat from ALL 4 food groups. Protein, Dairy, Fruits &

Vegetables, Grains plus some Oils & Fats

- Try to eat fruits & vegetables with every meal. It adds more fibre to your body and it makes you feel full on fewer calories.

- Increase water intake. Drink decaf tea, hot liquids, Stevia flavoured waters or drinks.

- Limit milk intake. Milk is essential, but I had a gorge fest with milk and it was one of my nemeses, so I limit myself to 2 glasses and that includes the milk in my cereal and tea. I often select yogurt as my milk choice.

- Find the time to cook at home and curtail eating out. I always broil when I can and invested in a kitchen grill. When dining out, always choose the healthy choices on the menu.

- Follow the rainbow; add green & colour to my diet in the art of salads, berries, veggies and fruits.

- Add nuts and fibre to my plate and my snacks. Walnuts and sunflower seeds add protein.

- Have a cheat day. Allow ONE grace period hour EVERY week to enjoy a treat. My choice is popcorn every Thursday night.

Just as everyone has their own individual story, everyone must find what program works best for them. Please understand that this works for ME and should not be taken as the regimen that you should follow or make you think that because it works for me, it will for you. I am positive that should you be experiencing the need to get healthy and the desire to change your lifestyle out of necessity for a happier and healthier future, perhaps some of my plan can be applied and start you on the right path.

The other key component of my weight loss success and an element missing in many people's journey to successful dieting results is EXERCISE. Without fail, there must be some form of physical activity every day. Walking, jogging, Zumba, dance fit, aerobics, swimming, cycling, weight training, canoeing, skating, chair exercises, martial arts, dancing, gymnastics, anything. You must find *your* mode of exercise but you must do SOMETHING and you need to do something physical at least 30 minutes every day. Follow the 10,000 steps rule.

Immediately, I recognized and accepted that my love affair with food was preventing me from having a love affair with myself. I needed to find MY mode of exercise. I was nearly 300 pounds, so a gym was not an option for me. I couldn't use the machines because I couldn't manoeuvre the Elliptical, and I couldn't physically endure fitness classes. The sanest choice for me was walking, mainly due to my obesity. I chose walking because it was easy, cathartic, and I could hum, sing, and talk to myself while enjoying the tonic of the crisp Canadian air, which I love. It made me feel better physically and psychologically and my body craved it. At first the routine was a challenge. I started out slow and ended up in sweaty clothes, but eventually the walks became less strenuous and I pushed for longer distances. I walked at least 45 minutes, which eventually turned into an hour. That roughly equals about five kilometres an hour. As my body got used to the exercise, the intensity of the walks increased. I did the bulk of my walking in the evening, after supper, which helped curtail my lifelong habit of eating at night. I also found a great buddy in my neighbour Deborah Harrington who accompanied me on the moonlit walks and stops at Tim Hortons for tea. Living in Canada, it also means that there are four really bad months of snow and ice, however, from the onset, I still got out and walked every day; rain or shine, snow or sleet, hail or storm. As the seasons changed I became addicted to the adrenaline of my body being exercised on a regular basis for the first time in fifteen years.

It is my stringent steadfast belief that my success has been mainly due to the fact that I got up and started walking. My routine now consists of walking an average of seven to ten kilometres every day and I make the effort to fulfill that quota every day unless thunder and lightning presents itself. I get out and take my running shoes on a journey anytime I can find the time; daytime, afternoon and evenings. I love to spend my weekends hiking throughout Southern Ontario conquering many nature trails, participating in fundraising walks, or sauntering on river side jaunts. Once I began controlling my eating habits and started walking, I have to say the results were almost immediate. It was as if the fat was jumping off of me, leaving greasy splashes on the pavement behind me as I was walking. *"Ker-plunk and Buh-bye!"*

Of course, walking every day isn't the only thing I do. As my story unfolded, I gradually added more exercise to my lifestyle. Obviously, my fitness regimen includes taking and teaching several Zumba classes per week. I also love to bike ride as much as I can and attend a weekly Boot Camp class with Gladys Knier. While maintaining a daily common sense eating plan; I do SOME form of fitness EVERY day! I have set realistic long-term goals to stay fit and to stay on this pattern. My weight should stay off, as long as the lifestyle changes I have made remain. **Healthy Eating + Exercise = Success.**

God gave me a second chance; I embrace it every day and never take it for granted. Being fit is my choice and my doing, as being unfit were my choice and my undoing. Big Sir granted me penance and a new way to be free. I get outside every day and thank HIM every day and make sure that my days are filled with paying it forward and never stopping my quest for betterment. I love my life, I love who I am and I get a kick out of being Joan Minnery. When you've stared down a gurney in the E.R. and have seen what the future holds, you have ONE choice. Give IN or get UP and give it all you've got! In other words, *"Put Down The Fork And Get Moving!"*

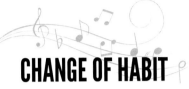

CHANGE OF HABIT

"It is time for us to stand and cheer for the doer, the achiever, the one who recognizes the challenge and does something about it."
- Vince Lombardi

My life had always been lived on the frontlines, battling a war against fat. I've been up and down and way up and way down. I've been a size ten and I've also been a size twenty six. I've tried ALL of the plans, all of the diets, all of the fads and all of the gimmicks. YES they worked, all of them, but my weight loss never seemed to last. I always ended back in the drive-thru line ordering a fish fillet. It seemed that once I became thinner there was always a reason (generally a jerk) that started me back up on my climb and another descent into weight gain Hell.

I used to wake up every Monday morning saying, *"Today is the day I'm going to lose weight,"* and then by noon I ended up in the drive-thru ordering a milkshake, fries and a greasy hamburger. Tuesdays turned into the day that I wished I had listened to myself the day before, so I would end up defeated. I beat myself up and lamented in the fact that I had messed up again. I would then convince myself, *"I'll start next week."* The same pattern occurred over and over again; week after week, month after month, year after year, pound after pound after pound.

I needed to change my thought process. When I started my journey on August 27, 2010, I did not say, *"Today is the day I'm going to lose weight."* Instead I looked in the mirror and said, *"Today I CHOOSE TO LIVE."* It all came down to making choices that were affecting my entire existence and if I wanted to stay here, I had to stop making those choices and Choose *Life!*

When I started my weight loss journey, I set my goals on the short term and fantasized about the long term. Initially, I was only attempting to get through the first three weeks unscathed. Once I passed that threshold, I set my sights on reality. I envisioned what life would be like a year from that moment. I set out on a realistic effort of a one year sabbatical from the life I presently knew. I put forth a question to the universe, *"What will I look like one year from today?"* One year; just 365 days out of a 44 year life. Time flies by so quickly; surely I could commit to ONE year! I was worth it; I knew that BJ certainly was and I knew that if I didn't do something now that there would be no more chances; it would become too late.

With this in mind another one of my catchphrases became, *"Imagine where you will be one year from today."* I had to get a mindset, a total selfish ego enhanced mindset that this is about ME and nobody else. It's a full on commitment of time. It took me decades to get to where I was in August, 2010 and I knew full well that it was going to take *two years* to get the weight off safely and healthily. It seemed daunting; I was faced with the thought of a 24 month battle. *That had to change.* I had to change that thought process *immediately.* Resetting my brain to stop calling it a battle and refer to it as a journey allowed me to start looking ahead to two years of junk food sobriety and two years of a total lifestyle change, setting realistic, attainable goals.

Did I know? Did I have any idea? Was I able to visualize what I would look like? How I would feel? How others would view me? Did I conceptualize ANY of it? No. I am glad that I did not know because the happy onslaught of positive changes and the constant gifts that continually blessed my life would not seem as sweet. I didn't start to be thin, I started to be well. I have done a cornucopia of weight-loss programs before with mixed results. This journey has been vastly different simply because I refused to focus on losing weight. My desire needed to be maintained with this firm belief: to be healthier.

Like many of us, I've always placed far too much emphasis on getting to a certain weight and watching the scales closely. My commitment was to stay focused on getting fit and obviously my weight loss came with that. For me, that meant not making the scale my priority. It meant knowing that I was eating better, that I was moving along with the newfangled experience and the euphoria of new clothes, and increased physical happiness. It was important for me to conceptualize that I was eating better and devoted to changing my health and wellness schedule. What was happening on the scale wasn't the key component of my journey. It was what was happening to me inside, physically, emotionally and spiritually that helped me change Fat into FIT!

"I did it my weigh."

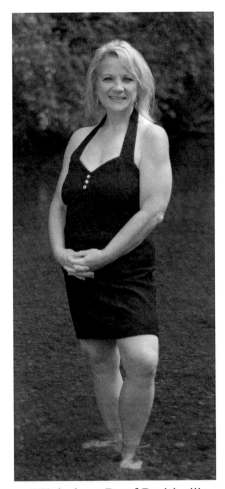 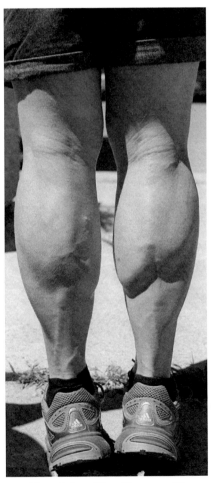

FITabulous Proof Positive!!!   Repairing The Damage!!!

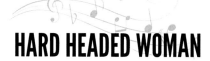

HARD HEADED WOMAN

Being strong doesn't mean you always have to fight the battle. TRUE STRENGTH lies in being able to walk away from all the nonsense with your head held high.

I was asked for years, *"Why are you fat?"* And after my weight loss, people asked me, *"Why were you fat?" "How come you took so long?" "If you knew HOW to lose weight, why didn't you?"* Part of my endless crusade in speaking in front of audiences, writing a book and being so public about my battle has been to educate the general public and others battling the demon about the reasons behind weight gain, the failures of weight loss and the truths surrounding the reason people eat. It was also paramount to make a valiant effort to dispel the misconceptions that the average person has towards obese persons and the realization of why people are fat. The myth out there that overweight folks are simply lazy and spend their lives sitting on couches slobbering down calories couldn't be further from the truth. The majority of the people I know are not skinny nor are they sporting slim physiques. There isn't a person within the hundreds of amazing people I know whom I would characterize as lazy. In fact, they are unequivocally the direct opposite. While their food choices may be in question, their lives are fruitful with rewarding careers, family, and home/leisure activities. I will proudly state that prior to my weight loss, I was one of the busiest people in our home town. There are infinite *other* reasons people are overweight and what needs to be understood is in that -- understanding!!!

Yes, it may be true that some folks just like food. There are many out there that really enjoy their consumption and their love affair with food. What needs to be understood is their addiction to the taste of the foods they are choosing is exactly like a heroin addict's high, a smoker's nicotine necessity and a drinker's euphoria. It is an addiction, be it to sugar, salt or perhaps the addiction to the pleasure one attains from eating. There is a sense of entitlement one gives to oneself in salivating over chocolate or a bag of chips or a fruit laden ice cream. It makes us feel good. It allows us to escape. It provides us with an instant reward in the mind.

There are a lot of misinterpretations out there about WHY people are overweight or why people continue to eat when they know they are unhealthy. How many times have many of you heard this insensitive question, *"Why are you fat?"* Let's face it -- we are fat because we overeat, plain and simple. However blunt that may be, we all understand the reason we are fat. We eat and we gain weight. What should be focused on are not the reasons we are fat, but the reasons we are eating. The question needs to be changed into something understandable and identifiable. Fat is the outcome of our overeating. WHY Do We Eat?

So what was my reason? Let me be totally frank. I love food. I enjoy eating. There is one reason that I was fat, and that was because I was a hefty eater and chose to continually put high caloric fat laden food down my gullet. As a carb addict, I love the taste of salt and when my mouth was tantalized it was an insatiable glutton fest; I had to have more. I ate like a pig in a sty, fast and furious and without breathing. I am a voracious eater with a huge appetite. Anyone who has sat with me throughout pot lucks and buffets knows I can pack it in. I eat very quickly and have large plates. I used to inhale my food and basically put my head down and didn't come back up for air until I was done. I suffered from gluttony at times, as there seemed to be an endless pit. I gobbled food up at record speeds, almost as though I was in constant fear of it being taken away for me. After all, so many people and things had been taken away from me. To rationalize and explain it, my lack of love was replaced with bowls of chips, handfuls of candy or cans of pop, yet the bottomless pit was never satisfied. I was never full. It was never enough because inside I was empty. It was this emptiness that was eating at me, plain and simple. Ultimately, there really is a great deal of truth to the familiar limerick, "It's not what you're eating; it is what is eating you." I had to find out why I was eating like I was.

Some of the reasons I was eating are all written within the pages of this novel. There were others such as financial woes, job loss, elderly parents, teenage rebellion, fear, betrayal, loss of friendships, life plans not working out, health scares; the list is endless. I was unhappy and didn't like my life. No matter how successful I appeared, the truth is that I had given up on my career, and I lost my way. I had no base line for my self esteem. My resolve to deal with stress had bottomed out. My self esteem had bottomed out. My health was suffering. I did not care. Everything about me was hurting. I felt insignificant.

Food became my locked door to the future. It became my albatross around my neck and three chins. It became the hoards of cellulite on my upper thighs. It became the belly overhang and fat on my arms. It became my body odor. It became the extra hair growing on my face. It became the sloppy clothes. It became the expensive wardrobe at the fat lady store. It became my humiliation. It became ME. Eating was my coping mechanism. Eating was how I learned to COPE. The biggest coping skill I had was stuffing my face, although cope came to stand for *Cannot Overcome Personal Emotions*. It was how I learned to live. It became my way out. It became my only alternative to the pain in my heart. I learned to replace the lack of love in my life with an abundance of food. Nobody would love me, so I had a love affair with the fridge. Food became my best friend for life. Well folks, my BFF nearly killed me!!! I had to deal with the pain. It was THIS which presented the deepest test on my ability to cope and continue to be successful. Only through walking, meditation, talking, praying and sitting on a lawn chair was I able to finally isolate myself enough to face my demons and deal with my emotions.

Having said all of that, there was an obvious necessity in my life that had to change; something pressing that needed to happen to achieve success and to maintain equilibrium. Losing weight became the easy part, eliminating the negative cause brought about an unexpected battle. In order to find me and find my happiness again, there needed to be changes and some of them came with a heavy price, but I was willing to pay it. BJ needed his mom back and she was gone. I had to do *everything* in my power to help bring her home from that road of destruction. It was that path on which I almost perished, but that rocky path evolved into the symbol for the Rock of Strength & Ultimate Survival. I had to save Joan. I was on a life saving mission to preserve MY life and the life of my son. HE is the only one I cared about and at all costs whatever it took to keep BJ's Mom *alive*, it was done. I was willing to do whatever was needed in order for me to get well. It no longer mattered about friendships. It became a life preserving mission and if that meant that chambers of my heart had to be closed off to get me well -- so be it.

Over the course of the first year of my journey, I began clearing house of all negativity in activities, surroundings and people. When I am asked why certain folks are no longer in my life and why I walked away -- it was for my son. It doesn't mean that my feelings for those people changed. My deep appreciation never stopped for what they once meant in my life and what they may have done for me during our times together. It became about the here and now. Anyone that didn't foster that mission or created negativity, in attempts to cause me to steer off course was deleted. If certain friends were entangled in a web that was set to destroy me, they too needed to be removed. Whatever cost, nobody was safe from elimination, whatever was deemed necessary and whoever needed to go, all bets were off. No holds barred, no friendships were safe. Who needed to go -- went. You get in my way -- OUT!!!

Would I change *anything* that I did to accomplish this goal? *Hell NO!* These events unfolded in a way that was necessary and what needed to happen was supposed to happen. I had to save myself from my own self and my own inner destruction. The walking melded into the metaphor of walking away. Walking wasn't just about fitness, it was about *freedom*. Complete freedom and total mental clarity and enabling me to not only *feel free* but for my body to *be free*, and that meant my mind and my spirit. In order to achieve success and better my health I had to walk away from some very tender pieces of my heart. Truth be known, dieting and fitness became easier as time went on; walking away was the hardest and most difficult part of the journey.

Joyfully walking away paved for a new foundation and much needed period of solitude. A vast amount of people within my former life and inner circle were gone. I needed that alone time to heal, to get well, to write, to read and to focus. That solitude enabled me to cement my own strength and resilience. I will always maintain that what happened had to happen; it was exactly perfect. When a door is shut, a new one always opens; sometimes they *swing open!!!*

My chosen "go to place" had always been App's Mill; however, it always ended in me sitting on the rock and eventually self destructing into a puddle of pity party tears. I had tried to walk and heal at App's Mill, yet the painful realization was that there was too much pain associated with that spot. On a Saturday afternoon in late May of 2011, I decided to re-route and go through the town of Paris. I ended up going on a long drive through the countryside and somehow just happened to wind up on the east side of the Grand River near the train bridge. I had the windows open and Randy Travis blaring on the stereo. I heard the water. I saw the scenery. I saw the dam and I immediately stopped my van. I sprinted up the escarpment and found my new paradise. It's the canoe launching area, but I affectionately refer to it as Loni's Lookout, taken from a madcap play that I was in where I had the role of a Loni Anderson type of character. Loni's Lookout became my new perch. This new place echoed freedom. I was out in the open above it all, on the path overlooking the Grand River and listening to the water. Loni's Lookout is my haven and the nuance of every positive aspect of my journey. Up on that perch at Loni's Lookout is where I started writing this book.

BOSSA NOVA BABY - ZUMBA

When God closes a door, He opens a window. In my case, He opened up every single window on a skyscraper. There's a famous saying that reads, *"The road to Hell is paved with good intentions."* Well I'll tell you one thing: the road to Heaven on Earth is certainly paved with a Zumba class. *Hell hath no fury like a former fat woman with a license to teach Zumba!!!*

By the spring of 2011 an out of the blue unexpected gift of enhancement was dropped on me. Enter the Art In Motion Dance Studio (AIM) on Brantwood Park Road in Brantford. AIM is owned by my high school buddy, Brian Sloat and his wife Kelly. She telephoned me to congratulate me on my success; she and Brian had been reading about it on Facebook. Kelly relayed that they had been so inspired by my story and due to their happiness for me, that they would like to become a part of my journey. They graciously invited me to come and try out a Zumba class at their studio. Walking into AIM Studios on April 25, 2011 is parallel to the moment that Dorothy goes from black & white in Kansas to colour in the Land of Oz. My thoughts on AIM were immediate, *"All sorts of fabulous characters combine together in joy and merriment and all there for one purpose, to get fit through dance."*

Through the doors of AIM was something unique, magical and vastly different from my norm. There was a friendly welcoming atmosphere that breathed total, encouraging family support. AIM was parallel to finding nirvana. There were no pre-conceived notions of who I was or who I am, they didn't know me prior to my arrival and only knew THIS Joan. They didn't know the fat, depressed lost victim I was formerly. All they knew was this phoenix that had

75

risen. I was among my peers with like-minded individuals who just wanted to dance and shake away the cobwebs of their day for an hour or so. I made friends very quickly and with that, my social life improved exponentially. I had finally found a place where I fit in.

Up until I started at AIM, my fitness life had only been walking. I knew that I had to start kicking it up a notch, as I had hit somewhat of a plateau. Once I added in the intensity of Zumba and Dance Fit, my weight once again started to fall off and my body began to firm and tone up. I finally had a figure to show off, not just a skinnier face. Zumba is contagious and it gets under your skin, leaving you with the lustful feeling of wanting more. I am addicted to the music, the camaraderie, the dance moves and the total body workout that it provides. I had forgotten the intoxication of Latin music after being away from the Dominican Republic, where I'd spent 2 years. It came back at me with a vengeance. Old familiar beats were back in my hips, my thighs, my legs and my happy twinkle toes were matched by the humongous smile on my face. The girl that got lost somewhere absolutely rekindled and got her groove back.

I cannot highlight enough how AIM has had an overwhelming impact upon my whole weight loss and self transformation. I became a permanent fixture in the fitness classes, being hailed affectionately as the "woo hoo!" girl. I merrily joined AIM's Latin performance dance team and we started performing at several events around town. I also braved their grueling once a week 3 hour Zumba boot camp which lasted for 2 months enabling me to take my body to a 90 pound loss.

Due to both the success of the Boot Camp and my motivational presentations taking off; Kelly and Brian approached me about implementing a 90 Day Weight Loss and Fitness Challenge at their dance studio. We opened up the participation to studio members and then to the public. Through the help of the Boot Camp and my Facebook illustriousness, we sold out the challenge on the *first* day, and so began my life as weight loss counsellor and running my own weight loss group. Our group met every Wednesday with our participants uniting together to weigh-in, take part in the weight loss discussions, workout and strive towards healthier excellence. It was directly due to the success of our program at AIM that prompted Nancy Good to invite me to start another weight loss group at Tranquility Place Residence, which was supported by Kelly and Brian.

The year of 2011 was a super duper year. By December I had lost 105 pounds and my transformed body had dropped 10 dress sizes. I gained an abundance of energy and happiness that was exuding from my shrinking body. I woke up every morning wanting to shout *"Hallelujah!"* Then the most incredible occurrence sailed directly towards me, invigorating me to even greater heights. After being trained by Kelly Sloat, the master of them all, I was encouraged greatly to pursue a dream of mine to get back into teaching fitness and become a Zumba Instructor. Alongside Brian, I obtained my Zumba Instructor certification license on December 3, 2011. After that, Kelly gave me the absolute highlight of my Zumba love fest, when she asked me to demo a song on Wednesday, December 28, 2011 at AIM. It was the calm before the storm.

As everyone knows, I'm a massive Elvis fan. In fact I'm not just a fan, I'm downright eccentrically nuts about him. I've had quite the colorful life in the Elvis tribute world and when it came time for me to choose my coming out song; I knew exactly where I was going to go -- to the KING himself! One song in particular kept resonating in my head, Bossa Nova Baby. Much to my delight, there was a funkier techno revamped version of it that just screamed *"PICK ME"*. So, with my Elvis dance moves career behind me and a definite knack for doing things outlandish, I put together a three minute in-your-face, high intensity, invigorating Elvis Zumba love routine. I presented my Zumba number to the mainstays of AIM and in return received an outpouring of immediate smiles, enthusiasm, sweat, fun and accolades of *"You Go, Girl!"* There was no stopping me.

And So The Zumba Crazy Train Began...

Brian and Kelly offered me a job at AIM. I had been running the weight loss group but they knew my dream was to teach Zumba. They asked me teach one night a week in a tag team class with my new found gal pal, Linda Kuntz. What a brilliantly high spirited, fun filled and sometimes silly class. We combined the 90 Day Challenge with our Zumba class and this is where Keith Curley danced his way into the AIM family and ultimately into my arms (More on this later).

That winter I began instructing at two other locations in Brantford. My other Monday night weight loss group was in full motion, so we agreed to adopt the same plan we were doing over at AIM. The ladies loved it and became instantly well-versed in the songs and movements, all while jamming out to the Latin beats and the sexy moves. I also started teaching Zumba at the Academy of Dance, another dance facility in Brantford. During our first night, we were abounding with people who just kept walking in and taking a spot on the dance floor. While I knew a few of them, most of them were strangers who had heard through the cyber grapevine that I was leading a Zumba class and had come to be Zumbafied! As word got out, there was a surge in the number of attendees. I knew I had hit a grand slam. This was cause for celebration and also caution, due to the fact that while we enjoyed our location at the Academy, it was obvious from the onset that we would need to start looking for a gymnasium to house the bodies. We initially moved to Christ the King School and thoroughly enjoyed a packed house in their gymnasium, which began as a fundraiser for a school project. That success then manifested itself into both the Catholic Women's League from St. Basil's Church and St. Mary's Church approaching me about beginning Zumba within their facilities. Our classes were being attended by many of the same women and men and a network of enthusiasts soon began following me to all locations.

Why is my Zumba so successful? Zumba is huge everywhere. Anyone who teaches welcomes their own degree of prosperity. I believe my individual good luck is due mainly to the fact that not so long ago, I weighed close to three hundred pounds and couldn't get through a minor dance routine without heart palpitations and the onset of angina sweats. Many of the people I am leading are also embarking on their own individual health and wellness journeys; they seek validation and motivation through me. I used to be one of them -- I used to be the one that needed the push to get going. When I started Zumba at AIM I was feeling awkward and self-conscious about my weight. I was the biggest person in the room, yet I always lovingly obtained my push from Kelly and their other instructor, Lauren. What a beautiful example of "come full circle" that I have been able to continually pay forward by returning their kindness to others. My Zumba peeps are a high-spirited group of women and men who are dedicated to educating themselves to lead healthier lives and gain some insights into how to enhance them through basic natural weight loss and exercise.

I love teaching these FITabulous people. It's an absolute tonic to be their leader and to offer a sense of encouragement and proof that you can turn your life around and make a change for the better. What a blessing for me to be up there coaching them through Latin dance and funky rhythms while spurring them on with my huge big blue eyes and a smile as large as Memphis itself. I cannot thank Brian and Kelly Sloat enough. I owe *everything* to them. In this book, they are the heroes.

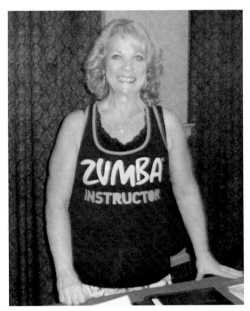

Having More Fun Than One Person
Should Be Allowed To Have!!!

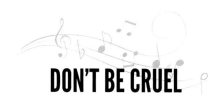

DON'T BE CRUEL

The journey to 150 pounds didn't start off all sunshine, lollipops and rainbows; in fact quite the opposite. There is a lot of hatred out there towards fat people, and those who suddenly try to get slim or go out in public are often met with a great deal of ridicule. Let's travel back to the winter of 2010. I was out for an evening stroll along Charing Cross Street in Brantford, just in front of the Nan King restaurant. I was en route to my sister Anne's house. I was silently boasting that I had just passed the KFC restaurant, which was a place I used to frequent often. During my private victory party I crossed the street onto the curb and suddenly got pelted with something on my left shoulder. As the object ricocheted off of my arm, I realized that a group of teenagers had just driven past me and hurled a fresh, hot Tim Hortons coffee at me. I began to feel the heat inside the left arm of my pink winter coat which was saturated and stained. Having a hot coffee hurled at me did hurt and it frightened me. I picked up the cup and the lid (which had flown off), carrying them both to my sister's house. Upon arrival, she was in utter astonishment as I showed her my wet sleeve along with the remnants of the coffee. The incident left me forlorn for a few hours. I never cleaned that stain off of my coat, using it as constant reminder of my journey.

Sadly, that wasn't an isolated incident as a few months later; I also got brandished with a full water bottle just a few blocks up from the same spot. It was obviously aimed at my head. Now in fairness, I only assume that these incidents happened because I was a fat lady walking. True enough, older teenagers who are merely out looking for something to do have the capacity to be total blockheads; however as a person who has faced it my entire life, I'm not going out on a limb to bet that if I had been a slender woman out walking, that wouldn't have taken place. I can lay claim to this because once the weight came off and I continued my walking regimen, I have yet to receive even one negative comment from any peanut gallery in town!

Some of the worst atrocities occurred at traffic lights with middle-aged men saying horrible fat comments as I was crossing the street. I will never fully comprehend the cruelty of cowards taking pot shots at a large-sized stranger. There is a sad bitterness of being out in the sun, care-free and doing something positive, only to have some clod just look out his window and bellow, *"LOSE SOME WEIGHT!"* I have always attributed this phenomenon to men being angry with their mothers or wives and not being able to say anything to them so they say it to strangers instead.

Of course, men weren't the only culprits. I've also had my fair share of car loads of women hauling insults as I was walking while being jury and executioner. If you think that people don't still say *"Tubbo," "Fatty,"* or other despicable names; think again.

Ironically, one of the many cross walk attack insults occurred in front of McDonald's on King George Road in Brantford. What was brilliant for me is the fact that instead of walking straight in to drown my sorrows in calories, I continued on another 40 minutes fighting back tears that eventually turned into pride. That seems to be how I handled the many adversities, the ones that came at me, always seemed to spur me on with more desire and gusto. The more that was thrown at me (both literally and metaphorically) the more the fire burned under my feet.

When you are almost 300 pounds and you suddenly start putting yourself through an intensive walking program, there's bound to be residual side effects. Six months into my journey, I developed a nagging knee complaint, which I have attributed mainly to the direct impact fall in Delhi. I got sidelined from walking for 6 weeks as a Baker's Cyst had developed along with a torn muscle. The walking brought the injury to the forefront and sadly will always be a continual source of woe.

Of course there is also the never to be discussed in public

humiliation of the main side effect of dieting, especially when you had 300 pounds of fat on your person. That fat is going to sag; it's going to hang and it's going to be unsightly. There is no tightening beyond a certain point. Once you've lost weight, what you see is what you get, unless you opt for surgery. I've had to learn to live with saggy skin on my arms, my breasts, my inner thighs and the all too real continual reminder of the tummy hang. I embrace it; it's with me as a constant reminder of where I used to be and how far I have come. I call mine, my *"Oscar."*

Despite all of the above adversities, I was not prepared for one of life's most prolific lessons. I could never have predicted the all too familiar realization: *You Want To Find Out Who Your Friends Are NOT — Lose Weight.*

As I have learned from being so much in the public eye; you have to have a *very* thick skin to survive in the entertainment business. Putting oneself out there can often result in being fodder for the naysayers and open you up as prey for ridicule. There is *always* going to be someone who wants to crap in your cornflakes and cause negativity. For every 100 fans, you get 10 folks that think you suck. For every bash you receive, you receive 100 accolades. I will never understand humans; they can be so bitterly vicious towards one another.

Sadly with my weight loss journey, I also faced the very unsettling realization that my weight loss success had garnered some negativity. It did not seem that everyone was happy about my new healthier attitude and my new love affair with myself, nor were they keen on me spreading my message of health. My new found strength also paved the foundation for my resolve in having to deal with some unexpected negativity that came at me like an out-of-control wild fire sparked by a tornado of jealousy and sheer bitter evil.

Some folks misunderstood that my journey was not just about the amount of weight lost and the number of pounds that have been taken off. My personal story was never simply about the transformation of my body; it was about the total life transformation which affected my entire personality, my heart and my soul. *How can it be negative to have a new strength and love for myself; a new inner self confidence and belief in myself?*

Prior to getting healthy, negativity was all around me and I was caught in the nucleus of a dark aura. I had become lethargic, lazy, cynical and I hated the world around me. Inside, I was still the same Joan who wanted to save the dolphins and prayed for world peace, but there was a hateful outer shell which had become very unlikeable. Yes I was still Joan, I still sang and taught music, and ran events and still cared deeply about those who were within my heart, but I was not happy. Moments of smiles and laughter occurred but they were only fleeting. I had 3 chins, I was a morbidly obese woman whose face looked at least 15 years older and I had chronic fatigue that showed on my frame and within my entire spirit. I was almost 300 pounds and going into a size 26, I had given up and had let myself go. I spent the better part of my days moping around, feeling sorry for myself, sitting on my computer chair waiting for any recognition from the outside world that I mattered. To put it bluntly, I had morphed into a fat, lazy oaf who ate non-stop, who didn't care about herself and sought some form of acceptance through insane means of validation. THAT person no longer exists. THAT person will never again see the light of day. THAT person had a few people around her that were comfortable with whom she was and had grown accustomed to her being unhappy. THAT person was seriously ill, physically and mentally. Sadly, had some of my associates been true friends, they would have recognized how dire things had become and instead of condemning me for changing, they would have fostered and embraced the change, allowing me to do whatever was necessary for me to become healthy. Their friend was on the brink of disaster, teetering on a cliff and needed assistance to be pulled back to safety. Instead, I found out rather shockingly, some were wishing to have the final push. Weight loss sabotage pounded ferociously on my door, which may surprise a great many people as I've been overwhelmed with a well documented legion of supporters. My saboteurs sprung up like cancerous growths from my former circle of life. Through human nature and plain old jealousy, they took great strides to try to knock me down and diminish my success.

I had taken the necessary steps to get healthy and as my

journey continued, my pants started to become saggy. I started to giggle more. My health factors which were affecting my life began to take a back seat to the overwhelming need to take another trip to the grocery store to buy more bananas. My smile broadened. I began to gain more confidence in myself and my energy levels skyrocketed. On a regular basis, I was walking along the streets of my neighbourhood and folks started rooting me on. As I continued to push forward in my running shoes, I also started to mentally work through years of damage that I had done to myself. Humming became a noticeable side-effect. With every step I felt the weight not only falling off my behind but also off of my shoulders. I felt great, I looked great. The scales were shouting *"GO GO GO!"*

I began posting the happy results on Facebook and Twitter and gathered an arsenal of well wishers. The world around me started applauding. My excitement cheered me on to purchase a new wardrobe; including my first ever jeans without an elastic waist! Coming into the new millennium, I also reinvented my Dolly Parton hair into a modern hairstyle. Two of my colleagues eagerly insisted upon a gift of a makeover and encouraged me to embody a sensual red number. It was the first sexy outfit I had worn in two decades. I was so delightfully happy with the results of the new me and the subsequent photo shoot, that I posted one of the pictures of me in the red corset on Facebook. Then all hell broke loose -- It was as if I had been convicted for a heinous crime against humanity.

For reasons unknown, a select few of my "friends" turned into sinister forces lurking in the background. They had taken quite a dim view of my weight loss journey which was catapulted to the forefront, showcasing their increasing displeasure about the makeover picture and subsequent progress photos I had posted on Facebook. Their repeated, spiteful, mean-spirited comments about the photographs evolved into a rampage much like a violent snorting bull over my "mid-life crisis." Facebook echoed an inundation of hateful laughs as they could not wait to see me gain back all of my fat and how they would delight in laughing at me more. The attacks became venomous and increasingly more loathsome. To add insult to injury there was also posted a cruel and insensitive animated photograph of a dancing elephant in jeans with her bottom wiggling. They had posted corresponding Zumba references relating directly to and poking fun at me, actually writing underneath the spinning graphic, *"Press the Dancing Elephant if you want to go to Zumba."* That post received chuckles and laughs. What I found perplexing is that this post on Facebook was liked and encouraged by mutual acquaintances that are morbidly obese themselves and from others who have people in their lives struggling with their own health and addiction battles. A great deal of attacks was then aimed towards my weight loss seminars and public speaking events. They referred to them as a joke, a good chuckle, that it was ridiculous and that I was pathetic.

My saboteurs wanted me to fail and they used cyber-bullying techniques in an attempt to derail me. Au contraire, it actually brought me even more success. The more they opened up their mouths, the more I closed mine. The more they spewed their hatred, the more I was determined to be successful. Their attacks on me did not deter me. In fact, what ensued was quite the opposite. An intense and positively energetic fire was lit under my feet. I became determined to pursue the dream even more than before. I knew that my struggle had been for the good and the betterment of my health and the overall positive future of my family.

While the sources were shocking, it's not uncommon for anyone who does something successful. I could chalk it up to being in the public eye, yet sadly human nature sometimes creates jealousy. Successful people are always going to have naysayers. I've learned over the years that those who may be with you as you start up the ladder might not be with you as you rise up the ladder and sometimes, they fall off and then start throwing rocks to knock you down. It's a sad state of human nature to want to knock someone down or wish for them to lose their footing and fail. How anyone could wish for BJ's mom to get ill again or deliberately set out to discredit me and ruin my support system through animosity and lies is totally baffling. I am truly sorry that a few of my "friends" collectively chose to spew hatred and brought others into their web of deceit and hypocrisy, but that just proved to me precisely who my *true* friends are.

One component of all of this is that I've had to learn and accept that their negativity towards my weight loss is *their* problem and not mine. It was never about me, it was about them. My very public and dramatic results have brought their fears to the forefront. I've inadvertently caused them to face their own unhealthy lifestyles, making them fearful of their own changes that need to be made. Change causes people to be fearful and fearful people strike out. Luckily, they also struck out in their attempts to ruin my success.

What is great about all of this is that while it was done to dissuade me, it actually propelled me up the ladder with gusto. It became the fire under my feet and the wind on my back to succeed. Hatred only fanned the flames for me to smile at the end of the journey knowing that I had done it through adversity and triumphed at the finish line. Actually, I thank them. I thank them for spewing, because it kept my eye furtively on the prize. It cemented my desire to win the battle. Truly, they were put in my path to destroy me, yet they inadvertently challenged my willingness, my desire and my compassion to love myself enough to be where I am today.

Yes, the naysayers DID make me stronger. And I believe that was part of the destined plan. While I was succeeding on my own, I did need an extra push, I needed to stay committed and focused. Once this all started happening, trust me -- not only did I stay committed, it became the major blessing in disguise for my resolve to be fearless. I may have started off with *"I'll show them,"* but it quickly turned into *"LOOK AT ME!!!"*

Perhaps to some the sight of an obese woman tackling Zumba made me look something like a dancing elephant. That's up to the beholder -- perhaps yes, perhaps no, but I'll say one thing that's for certain -- this dancing elephant is now laughing. *"WAIPA!"*

"You can break my heart, but I'll be damned if you're going to break my spirit." Anne Minnery

FREE

The pieces of me left
as peace came...

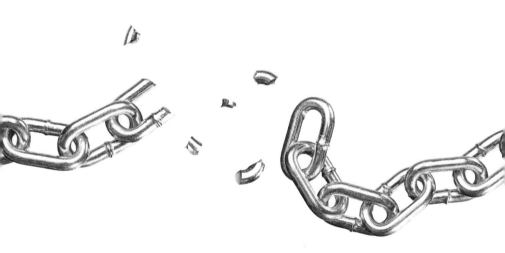

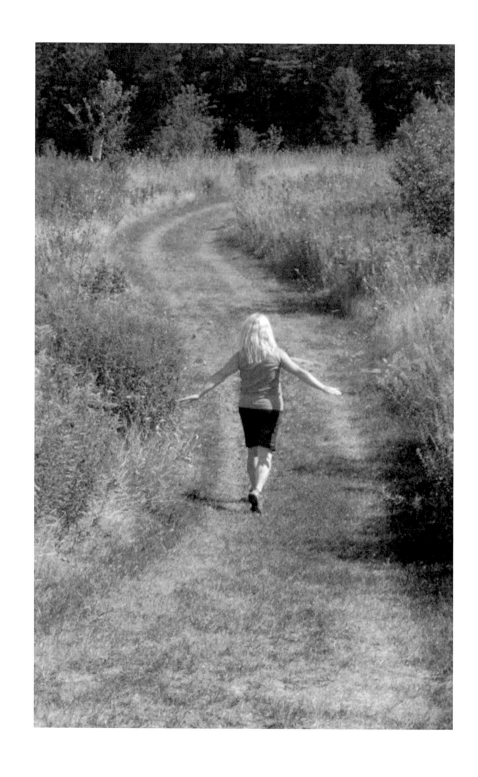

WHAT A WONDERFUL LIFE, THIS LIFE I'M LIVING – THE TRIUMPHS

Remember that amazing *Wide World of Sports* commercial that happily boasted the thrill of victory and the agony of defeat, showing sports clip highlights of thunderous wins and astronomical losses? While my weight loss was met with some degree of antagonism, those few strands of negativity paled in comparison to the tapestry of positivity.

Quite a few years ago, my mom asked my son what he wanted most in life. BJ's reaction was simple and ricocheted into my soul. *"I want to be able to put my arms around my mom again."* Earlier on in my journey, BJ went away for a week on a cruise with his buddy Brad Bridges and his parents. When he returned, I was waiting for him in the driveway of the Bridges' home in Mount Pleasant. BJ jumped out of the car, leaping at me without any forethought and threw his arms around me. *"Mom, I can hug you. You're getting little again."* THAT look on his face, as his long time wish had been fulfilled, along with the visible glee he was sharing, paved a new road for me and my steadfast incentive to keep on trucking.

I could write an entire book on the bounty of triumphs and victories with which I have been blessed since choosing to attain health and wellness. While boasting about the myriad of positive graces, I am certain I would inadvertently still miss numerous rewards, however, here are a few victorious "replays" from my weight loss journey.

After 2 months of weight loss, I was borrowing my parents'

car and pulling the seat belt over me. I was prepared to just put it under my armpit as I had for many years. Their seat belt never fit over my stomach. There was a sound in that seat that I had never heard before. I heard the seat belt click into place at first I didn't really take notice, but after a short second I wondered, *"What was THAT?"* I looked down and concluded that the seat belt had fastened, albeit snuggly. I undid the seat belt and did it again, repeating this sequence several times. One would have thought I had just composed my Opus. Believe me when I say, hearing that seat belt fasten into that buckle was as prolific as writing my own Oscar-winning original score. VICTORY!

As I became more ill, the alien attacks escalated from a few times per year, to every few months and eventually, they became a weekly occurrence. As my health improved, the pancreatic attacks that were happening weekly prior to August 2010 seemed to vanish. The acute vertigo which sent me to the medical clinic in Hamilton became a thing of the past. Migraines along with the nagging issues of dizziness and nausea dissipated. My endurance increased and my overall health went on a rapid incline. Memory and coordination improved while my thought process became clearer and functional. Continual comments were made about the appearance of my skin and how fluid it looked due to the constant feed of fresh air. Very few blemishes appeared and the outbreak of fever cold sores diminished. One side effect of eating well was that suddenly the heart-burn and late night acid reflux had disappeared. I used to inhale antacid pills. Shortly after the journey began, I noticed that the bottle hadn't been touched. There was only one answer to the why it hadn't been touched: I had changed what was curdling my stomach. VICTORY!

For many years, I could not wear fancy shoes on stage. I had to take them off because my feet were sore and couldn't sustain my 300 pound frame. I used to suffer horrifically from very painful, cracked and calloused feet -- they healed completely. After dropping the weight, I could wear high heel shoes and keep my feet covered. My number one fan and long time follower, Dorothy Hillgartner, happily boasted, *"Joanie, it's the first time I've seen you do a whole show with your shoes on!"* Speaking of shows, my voice became much sweeter and stronger, holding notes longer and with more sustenance and depth. VICTORY!

Feasibly, one of the ongoing happier occurrences came with the fact that I had to continually buy new clothes. As the weight was literally falling off of me, new clothing needed to be purchased on a regular basis. There is nothing more satisfying than grasping the fact that I was shopping for regular sizes at Wal-Mart and purchasing my first pair of jeans. While it became expensive, it was money feverishly spent with a Cheshire cat smile. Once I started shopping at the normal-sized clothing stores, there was an internal celebration of *free at last within* my soul. My once too-skinny clothes began to fit me again. I vividly remember leaving Pennington's for the last time, which caused me to choke up, yet I know that I quietly wished that I could go back to the store at midnight and moon it. Of course, there's the adverse side of this too. I had to throw out 7 bags of "fat lady clothes," some of which were brand new. It was a burden off of my shoulders even though it did sting to watch hundreds of dollars get stuffed into green garbage bags. The trade off was priceless. VICTORY!

In January of 2011, after years of flying on airplanes and having to sheepishly ask for the seat belt extender, I finally didn't need it. Of course, the added victory is that when I brought the food tray down it actually fit into my lap. At last, I was able to enjoy a meal with the tray down, not tilted upwards sitting on my belly with the possibility of having the food tray fall into the magazine rack, which had devastatingly happened before. Fitting into pants and dresses is one thing -- bringing that tray down into my lap: Priceless. VICTORY!

One of my plans of attack was to refrain from stepping on the scale. While I knew I was dropping a great deal of weight, I never knew exactly how much I had actually shed. In May, 2011, I finally braved the beast and placed my feet on the dog scale at the Fairview Drive Animal Hospital while waiting for Anne's dog Penny to be vaccinated. I rationalized that perhaps the scale would be large enough to hold me. At last I saw my weight -- it read 208 pounds. I did the happy dance. The last time I had seen my weight it read 283 pounds, and I morphed up much higher. The scene in the waiting room was an overly emotional one as I truly cradled the reality that I had lost an incredible amount of weight. VICTORY!

One of my journey's most euphoric moments is one that embraced my life in August, 2011. I was at Anne's home and guardedly stepped on the bathroom scale. IT HAPPENED -- I saw the number ONE at the beginning of the scale's numbers. I carried out the scale and presented it to my sister, holding the scale like a little girl holding her dolly. Anne looked at me. *"There's a one,"* I softly whispered. She looked at me inquisitively. *"Huh?"* Almost breathlessly I said again, *"Anne, there's a one."* She looked at my face, saw the expression in my dancing eyes, then looked at the scale. Her eyes welled up as she put both hands up to her face. We celebrated. I had hit the big ONE. It was the milestone I had been "weighting" for! For the first time in fifteen years, I had finally dipped below the two hundreds on the scale. As the song says "one is the loneliest number," yet to see that number finally say HELLO after such a long absence -- I embraced it as the GREATEST number!!! 'ONE-derland' was here. VICTORY!

In addition to the victories above, there were the obvious accolades from people as they saw the slimmed-down version of me for the first time. Sometimes people wouldn't recognize me or would walk past me with a double take. One woman at Wal-Mart asked me if I was Joan's daughter. Oh, the joy that day. VICTORY!

There was the euphoric night at McGonagall's Pub when my friends in the band BarCode (Jeff Harding, Les Posan Jr. and Andy McPherson) paid homage to me from the stage by dedicating and singing Elvis' tune, *Return to Sender*, with their own twist. Much to my surprise, they changed the words to "Return to *Slender*." Both Jeff and Les Jr. made memorable, tear-jerking stage endorsements and went on to congratulate and applaud me for the great job I was doing and the healthy message I was spreading. VICTORY!

Life took on an unexpected, sparkling new path when Mike Jennings, a fellow entertainer and battling weight defender, invited me to speak about my successful journey at his TOPS group. That engagement led to the inauguration of my motivational speaking career as I began to bring my story across North America while coupling it with female empowerment and turning people's lives around. VICTORY!

There was the shriek of happiness as I sat in a booth at Angel's Diner on King George Road and became instantly aware that my body actually fit behind the table in the booth. In previous years, I had to choose sitting in a chair, due to being crammed and uncomfortable. I sat down and there was space between my tummy and the table. Gone were the days of me sitting down gingerly and being leery of wooden chairs breaking or creaking. VICTORY!

I stopped needing to check the toilets everywhere I went in order to make sure I could use them properly, because certain toilets were either too high or too low for me to manoeuvre manageable and necessary cleaning routines. VICTORY!

Nobody will ever fully fathom the personal retribution of sitting in a bath tub and not feeling the overhang of my fat belly resting on my thighs that I had known for almost two decades. VICTORY!

Walmart again laid the concrete for another stepping stone as I was able to finally fit into size medium clothing and purchase a pair of thigh high boots and my first ever two-piece bathing suit. I hadn't owned a two-piece since I had a flat chest and was in Grade 3. There is no greater rapturous boost to the ego than to see one's self in a form-fitting spandex swimsuit. Of course, this is also parallel to being able to walk into La Senza to try on and purchase my first ever regular-sized bra and panties and yet another sultry bustier. VICTORY!

We had been performing at the Simcoe Fair on Thanksgiving weekend for many years. It was Monday morning of the 2012 showcase and I handed our regular sound guy the performance background tracks. He asked me who I was. He had no idea and had been doing our sound for almost a decade. VICTORY!

As I had been out walking pretty well every day around Brantford, I became a noticeable fixture on the sidewalks. An up swell of continual horn honks from passersby cheered me on. As I would stop for tea at Tim Hortons, the workers would encourage me. People would see me forging through the rain and post about it on Twitter. I will never forget the carload of St. John's students hanging out the window and clamouring, *"Keep Going!"* I also received waves from city bus drivers and city workers, in particular Derek Bateson and his crew, who made a point of giving me the smiling thumbs up, as they saw me on a regular basis. VICTORY!

There was a moment in 2011 when I was about to go out. BJ looked at me and I seemed to make him gasp. *"Mom you've lost so much weight. You're little; I never noticed that you're a little woman just like Nana."* His look of sheer acceptance was enough for me to continue on. I hope someday he'll tell his own children and instill in them the gift of health as he relays the story, *"Look what grandma did."* VICTORY!

In the winter of 2012, I received an unexpected email from Dahlia Gibson, the mother of two of my former vocal students. Dahlia graciously, albeit shockingly, informed me that she had written an original song about me and my journey. Dahlia is extremely slight in physique and gentle in nature, and while she couldn't empathize with my plight -- she explained that she had become so inspired and moved by my journey that she wanted to reach out and pay it forward to me, as I had been motivating so many others. One of my life's greatest gifts came to me in her composition, *The Sky is the Limit.* VICTORY!

On Sunday, August 26, 2012, after leaving a backyard party celebrating my 150 pound loss, BJ sent this text to me: *Hi Mom, I'm really proud of you and your accomplishment. I knew you had it in you; you're the greatest mom ever. I couldn't ask for better.* VICTORY!!!

In October, 2012, I received the prestigious honour of being awarded the Queen's Diamond Jubilee Medal for Health and Wellness Ambassadorship & Community Advocacy. This overwhelming award is presented to outstanding Canadians for their community service. VICTORY!

In the fall of 2012, I was nominated for Brantford's Best Fitness Instructor in the local Brant News Readers' Choice Awards. I won first place in the competition, which was followed by another award in 2013. VICTORY!

Due to my sometimes prevalent appearance in the local news, my success was accumulating a great deal of attention from the Brantford Expositor, the Brant News, Rogers Community

Television and other local media outlets. This in turn echoed into neighbouring communities such as Hamilton, London and Kitchener. People must remember my Elvis life with the Graceliners and Memphis Motion, gleaning a great deal of TV appearances on talk shows, news programs and within print publications. My eccentric professional life always welcomed a long-standing kinship with the press. Reports travelled quickly that the Big Elvis Lady had a new story to share. Via Facebook and Twitter, my success story started to get picked up by various websites, as supporters began submitting my name. *Shapefit.com* in particular became very keen on me and what I had to offer to their readers. They invited me to become join their team as one of their bloggers. They then asked permission to submit my name into a potential pool of weight loss success stories for various magazines, and that is how the *BIG DEAL* happened.

Everyone sees these magazines at the checkout counter in the grocery store. We all read the headlines, wondering if any of what they say is true. We second guess ourselves when looking at them, speculating about whether or not there are fake people on the covers of the magazines. Let me be the person to stop the guessing. Those people and those stories are real. In the December 2012 issue of the international magazine *First for Women,* I was featured on the front cover. It's a small picture of me on the bottom right hand corner, but I am there. I also had my story featured within the magazine as a role model for effective weight loss and the power of self love. That experience included a professional photo shoot with my own make-up artist, hair stylist, wardrobe consultant and a two hour glamour shoot with Brantford master, Paul Smith, from Photohouse Studios. It was a girl's dream come true. VICTORY!

And finally....

It was the end of May, 2012 on a Wednesday afternoon. I was walking over the West St. Bridge and in the parking lot of the church, there was a man standing against his car holding a bouquet of flowers. He was a nicely dressed incredibly handsome man, leaned up against his car with brightly coloured orchids. I have to admit, the sight of this man with the flowers stopped me in my tracks. I immediately thought to myself, *"That guy is standing there to propose to somebody; how romantic; wow, lucky lady!"* I continued walking and then did a double take as I began to acknowledge who the man was but due to a vast change in his appearance, I couldn't quite place him as it was all out of context. I continued further, suddenly coming to the happy conclusion that the lucky lady was in fact me. Standing there against the car, all dressed up was my precious friend, David Griffin. Dave is a real estate agent for Century 21. He is also the lead singer for the band Hairy Mulligan, married to his equally gorgeous wife Sylvia and is a devoted dad. I shyly asked, *"Are those for me?"* Dave had this gallant smile on his face. He came towards me with one arm outstretched and the other with the huge bouquet. He bent down and gently hugged me. *"I was hoping to catch you. I saw you at Tim Hortons and rushed into Floral Express. These are for you. Congratulations on all of your success, I'm so proud of you."* I was gobsmacked. My heart skipped several beats, my knees buckled, my eyes filled and my mouth dropped. While fighting back his own emotions, he chivalrously handed me the flowers and got back into his car. It was a simple two minute gesture from a *true* Gentleman who wanted to pay respect to his friend. Tears were in abundance as I carried the flowers home, proudly displaying them in my hands while continuing my daily walking routine. I will never forget what my musical buddy did for me on that afternoon or what it meant to me as adversities suddenly vanished and transformed into triumphs. Dave's random act of kindness remains one of the most beautiful moments of any friendship I have ever known. VICTORY!

GOTTA LOTTA LIVING TO DO

As my healthy new lifestyle was emerging and having a dramatic positive impact on my whole catharsis, I also made relevant alterations to my professional career. My name is always going to be identified with music and I will always be a singer and an entertainer, yet, with my transformation came the epiphany that I needed to break free from the chains that were binding me down. My events and my career had become redundant and boring, if only to me. With so many changes occurring, it was a natural progression that my professional life was going to take an alternative route as well.

That's where my journey began to take on a life of its own. I have said it from the onset, there is a greater force driving my boat. It must be mentioned that this force shifted into warp speed once I found my way back to church at St. Basil's. Not preaching, just teaching.

I was craving something totally radical, new and exciting. As frightening as it may have been at first, I also knew that being scared of the future was sure as hell 100% better than looking back. I didn't know where I was headed, but I knew firmly what I did NOT want to do.

Being in front of thousands of people feels like home to me. It's where I find the greatest amount of joy and soul enhancement. I am no stranger to the spotlight. I love the stage and I thrive on making people laugh. On the advice of Bob & Marilyn Hajas, I began looking into the field of Motivational Speaking. They had given me the idea and had outlined the fact that I did this very type of presentation already and had been doing it for years as an emcee and the lead singer in my musical groups. They suggested that I combine my weight loss story with my music. I could sing and talk about myself, two things that I love to do!

I developed the trademark slogan *"Put Down the Fork & Get Moving"* and prepared my own motivational presentation about my weight loss journey including the raw honesty of the "A-HA" moment. Without warning, requests started coming in for me to come and talk. *"Whoa, hold on, I'm not even ready yet."* Although I wasn't truly prepared and had sea-legs about the whole concept, the calls started beckoning from various weight loss organizations and health and wellness expos. Groups were talking about my presentations and I got swept up with one appearance after another. It's been one Magical Mystery Tour that I never saw coming and I love every opportunity.

The next obvious phase in 'trimming the fat' as it were, was establishing a new direction with my music business and my performance life. I made a choice to walk away from the tribute business and cease putting on my own shows. My young protégé Alicia Skoretz and I stayed together as a duet after Memphis Motion disbanded. Alicia's equal pleasure in walking away shocked me as the effects of the team drama had also taken its toll on my young buddy. The stress of the hustle, bustle and insanity was gone and time was spent living life and being normal. We knew we wanted to stay together, but we also knew we wanted a new perspective. A new name was born -- *Touch of Sass*. It fit us both. While our voices and names will always be synonymous with Elvis and the '50s and '60s, it was a tonic to wipe the slate clean and start fresh.

We overhauled our entire show as we updated our look, our sound and our repertoire with songs from the radio hits of today. Alicia began attending karaoke with me on a regular basis to try out the new songs, and was eagerly as excited to also try out a new wardrobe. We could be girls; we could dress how we wanted. What a refreshing change! While we maintained our vast collection of songs and break into our former song bank all the time, we added some new upbeat country, pop, and Broadway collections. These changes opened up many new doors for us.

Alicia and I made a deal that we would tone down our

performance schedule, allowing more time for weekend fun. A few shows per month or every six weeks seemed agreeable. We also welcomed Taya and Kyra Humpartzoomian into the showcase, two long-time students of mine and veteran performers with Starr Sensations. Alicia's parents Larry and Laura are high school chums of Taya and Kyra's parents, Pam and Ty. Both families have been ardent friends of mine as we have shared many years of kindred musical spirits. Pam and Ty are two of my most cherished friends on the planet and I love their girls as if they were my own.

As for my own professional career, I am abundantly active as a vocal coach and direct children and teens in the Brantford Cabaret musical theatre group. I also welcome a steady stream of gigs with community groups, women's organizations, public concerts and senior residences. However, the performer now in front of them is hardly recognizable. There's a playful high-spirited woman dancing and thoroughly loving her craft. That transcends into the audience. I've got my MOJO working!

I Love The Person That I Have Become -- Because I Fought Like Hell To Become Her!

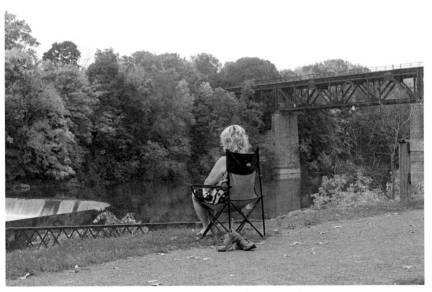

Loni's Lookout, Paris Ontario

I CAN'T HELP FALLING IN LOVE WITH FOOD

There was moment when I knew I would not fail, and I claimed it.

It's amazing how just a simple change in your appearance can have a resounding effect on most other aspects of your life. Self-confidence builds, you start to carry yourself in a different manner and you even start to talk differently, which may be in part, due to the other changes working together. Your body changes along with the belief in yourself. To be completely frank, a healthy body does work differently. A healthy body is full of vim and vigor and exudes positive energy. It releases all of that back into the bodily system. Keeping that in mind, a healthy body with a healthier state of mind gives you the power over yourself. Suddenly, you are in control and that control takes over every part of your being. What used to buckle your knees in despair now brings you to your knees in prayer.

I need to be perfectly blunt -- my battle is not over. I can never give up. While I am on a mission to never be where I was in August, 2010, I have to stay focused. I have to stay committed. I may have always proved that I am the little engine that can but I can never lose focus. Do I have bad days? Hell yes!! Have I gone off the rails? Yes. Life is happier. It is not perfect. I am healthier. I am not perfect. I am human. There are bumps in the road, and they are ok; it's part of weight loss. Sometimes, life just happens!!!

I have an addiction and I have a long life history of being unable to adequately deal with stress -- unless I am eating. I am an overeater and do have a horrific problematic dependency with food. Finding an alternative in how I deal with stress, was and will always be paramount to my survival. Addiction is always an addiction and mine has been hanging around for the better part of four decades. I cannot lull myself into a false sense of security. Life brings stress. Life brings issues. How do I fight the addiction? I've always been a firm believer that the answer to all demonic possession lies within the writings from one's psyche and within the locked compartments of the brain lay the truth behind the torment.

I have to be constantly vigilant. I have to remain committed to experiment with recipes, immerse myself in food education, attend seminars, surf the web, read, blog, journal and saturate myself in learning about proper nutritional foods and how they work and don't work for our bodies. Successful weight loss can only remain successful with a lifetime commitment to HEALTH. It is a lifelong commitment to the euphoria of freedom which has to remain militant and ever guarded. Addiction creeps back in, the demon takes hold and temptation is always there taunting and staking and tugging. My obesity is not cured. My addiction is not cured. I will never be cured, but I am free. No addiction is ever fully cured but it can be controlled. It can be defeated to the point of living freely with constant care and conviction of the knowledge of how to live with the addiction.

Food dependency needs to be controlled and monitored. I have been able to change what I am gorging on. Instead of feasting on nachos, chocolate bars and cola, I have been able to make healthier choices. I can now feast on large salads with fruit, nuts, chicken and yummy veggies and salad greens. I have found new tastes in olives, radishes, peppers, avocado, couscous, edamame beans, seafood, turkey, tuna, salmon, chicken, peameal bacon, beef and pork. I have found new ways to fill that bottomless pit. My sister and I tackled my food addiction with scrumptious outdoor BBQs on our mini-grill. We learned how to cook healthy and continue to enjoy various recipes. With her dog Penny in attendance; all three of us benefitted greatly. Anne even hopped on the band wagon in creating her own home made protein bars; which were quickly devoured by every sampler in Brantford resulting in baking orders.

Do I have pizza? Yes, but only a few times per year. I now

only eat two slices and don't reach for more. If I know I'm going to have it, I try to eat it earlier in the afternoon. I enjoy homemade pizza much more so that I can control what is on it. Do I still eat buckets of southern fried chicken? Uh, no, not buckets. Nonetheless I have had pieces on occasion. I must admit while it was delicious and memorable, I also know that particular brand of food is a major trigger for me. If I was a drinker, I wouldn't ingest liquor. So while I enjoyed the special treat, I knew that it wasn't something I would be trying again anytime soon. I choose to stay away. Do I have cheese flavoured nachos? I've had some small bags and enjoyed every bit. I also realized again, they are a trigger for my gluttony. They were the starring roles in my pity party foods. When I eat them I can easily be transported back to the rock at App's Mill. It's best to keep them in my past, along with my fat behind.

It's the old adage -- everything in moderation. Reducing my intake doesn't mean that I can never again have these foods, but for my sanity I just choose something else. My over eating was attributed to emotional disability, so why tempt fate if it's just easier to move away from the bowl at a party or sit elsewhere at a function?

Is my appetite still voracious? Yes, I'm still a big eater. I have learned to push myself away from the table and fill up on salads and protein. Desserts are something I seldom indulge in and if I do, I make a very conscious effort to make or take my own to a party. I'm not afraid of insulting anyone by bringing Angel Food Cake with me. In fact, it's quite respected. People understand it and they foster my necessity to be well.

While I love ice-cream, I have it in limited quantities. Although in the summer time, cones do appear within my hands a wee bit more than they should. I do my best to maintain militancy in what I choose to eat, when I eat, how much I eat and I monitor situations that can be hazardous. The battle still continues. Losing weight was actually the easy part; maintaining and keeping it off has been the chore.

I am still dealing with the demons and ironing out my emotions. Dealing with them can be just as much of a struggle as it is to not reach for the extra piece of cake or any slice for that matter. Pain is deep and sometimes outside influences still contribute to a slip. I still fight reaching for comfort foods. My refocus is in educating myself that while they may dull the pain and provide a ten minute respite of the mind; the food attributes to even more physical pain and anguish.

I soothe my addiction through finding alternatives. I make very conscious efforts to control my emotions through walking, bike riding and of course my Zumba classes. They are all great stress releases. I also do a lot of journaling and writing. I do crossword puzzles, write music, poetry -- anything to keep me busy. The cravings can often be diminished by moving away from the kitchen and opting for an herbal tea or a glass of water. If I find myself desiring something that I shouldn't be devouring, I make myself go for a walk. "Walk it off" applies in my case with optimistic gusto. It works. By the time I get a few blocks away, I'm transported into my happy reality. Plus, there are the added emotional highs I have been able to tap into by seeing all of the publicity, as I am inspiring others to the same. Now I feed off the positivity that my story has been having on others and the changes I have been able to inspire in other people's lives. To me, that adrenaline is comparable to a heroin injection. My food addiction has now transformed into an addiction of being fit and being healthy.

"I'm having more fun than one person should be allowed to have!!!"

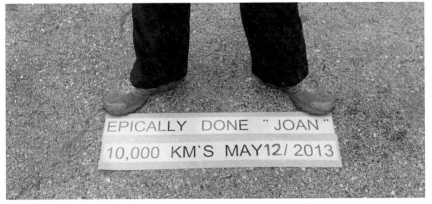

Over 10,000km and counting!!!

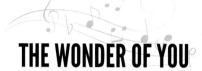

THE WONDER OF YOU

"When no-one else can understand me; when everything I do is wrong you give me hope and consolation. You give me strength to carry on. And you're always there to lend a hand in everything I do. That's the wonder, the wonder of you. And I'll guess I'll never know the reason why you love me like you do. That's the wonder, the wonder of you." - Elvis Presley, Words by Baker Knight

One of the main reasons for writing this book is that it is imperative that I pay it forward to the insurmountable amount of individuals who have been valuable components in my life and been positive influences throughout my entire restructuring phase. As for my gratitude accolades, there are many people to thank. In an endless scroll of people and organizations, there are far too many to mention. If I begin to list specific individuals I will inadvertently forget someone. I'd rather err on the side of caution.

For those of you, who have been a productive aspect of my journey, please know how grateful I am. I will forever be indebted to you. Without you, I could never have done any of it. When I started this journey, I did it for me and to get healthy. I had no idea that an army of support would surmount behind and beside me from like-minded people who were also suffering, nor did I have any comprehension of how the genuine compassion of friends and strangers would create an impenetrable chamber in my heart. With tears streaming down my face, in sheer happiness, I need to say, *"You know who you are. Thank You. Thank all of you very much!"*

For me, one of my main objectives in writing this is

forgiveness, mainly of myself, as I have allowed myself to apologize to me for making the decisions and choices throughout my life. My quest to be and prove myself right was interfering with the forgiveness I needed. Happily that dimmed as my mind's quest for clarity and serenity took precedence over everything else. I have found peace knowing that while sometimes detrimental, all of the people and events have had a purpose. There were reasons the events and relationships unfolded the way that they did. It was all a necessary part of the journey. In order for me to get to where I am presently, the climb had to be hard fought to enjoy the pay off in the end. I am so much sweeter now for having known the sour. I am so much more beautiful inside and out for having known the ugly. I am so much happier now for having known the sadness. I am so much more victorious for having known the defeat. I am so much more triumphant for having known the loss. I am healthier, happier, and to me *that's* all that matters. I made myself well again, in both body and mind. I have redeemed *justice* in my life. I got what I wanted, which was freedom and peace. I'm ecstatic to say that I've been de-stressed.

One of the key components to successful weight loss is accepting the blame for putting me in the precarious situation and admitting that *I* am responsible for allowing in the poison. I had to take the blame that I allowed food poison into my life and that I was directly responsible for allowing the poison into my personal life. I always had the control to change it, and I was the person who controlled it to keep on happening. I invited and accepted a certain caliber of persons into my heart and permitted them to assist in the damage; I was my own worst enemy. In turning my life around and becoming my own best friend, I was able to accept the responsibility and then do what was even more essential -- forgive. I was able to look myself in the mirror and say, *"I forgive you."* I allowed people to hurt me. I invited them in and allowed the abuse to continue. I lost control and belief in myself. I convinced myself I was not worth it, that I was nothing and settled for the same. I controlled what happened to me and it is my fault. I took blame and forgave myself. While forgiving those who hurt me is still a work in progress, I have been able to put it to rest and am seeking solace in the hopeful outcome of being able to confidently declare, *"I forgive you. All debts have now been paid."*

What very well may be the bigger testament here is the fact that I'm seeing myself and the world through a set of eyes that are alive, within a whole new Joan that never existed before. Every day I look forward to finding out what is next in store for me. What a revelation to be that positive about the future and to embrace the opportunities ahead. I have freedom. My body is free to exercise, pedal my bike, zip line, run down a hill, frolic through the woods on a trail, dance the waltz and wear high-heeled boots at a show. I can play baseball and run and catch a ball, I can do boot camp, I can do a plank, I can teach dance again. I am so proud of myself. The efforts were for me, the results are mine. Now my life sparkles so much I sweat glitter!

While the weight loss has been significant, what's more impressive is what I've gained. I've lost one hundred and fifty pounds and gained three times that in friends. There's a love story going on with me and those around me. People want to be around me as they are feeding off my positive energy. While I have a brand new fulfilling circle of exciting friends, many colleagues and former companions have come back into my life, which has been a tonic. Bev Miranda, my long time soul sister said it best, *"We have missed you. Welcome back Joan!"*

There is one person that could not go without a personal "thank you," and that's Anne, my little big sister. Her ferocious tenacity has always been the beacon of our family. Polio took the use of her legs from her at two years of age, yet she has travelled the world, held a government job and rose to heights higher than a thousand people could ever have attained collectively. She is forever my source of inspiration and true impermeable strength. While she may not have been physically able to walk with me; she has travelled every step of this journey with me. It is no secret that love had evaded me for most of my life, but I have been the ever accepting student of unconditional love from her. Anne was willing and did fight to the depths for me. There is no greater hero to me than the small pretty diminutive giant that calls me *"SIS"*

"Thank You, Thank You Very Much"

LOVING YOU – MY HAPPINESS!!!

While my personal relationships have always bottomed out, there is no doubt I have been blessed with one heck of an epic life. I have an amazing family, the greatest son on the planet, dear friends, a most unusual lifestyle of music, dance, fitness, performing and Elvis. Throughout all of this, as everyone knows, the one aspect of my life which has eluded me has been true love from a man. While I have accomplished every goal, travelled countries belting out tunes and dancing up wacky routines, love never came. I had resigned myself to a life of singlehood.

Turning my attention towards myself and getting healthy, I never gave up hope. I knew he was out there somewhere. I had so much to give and was willing to wait. I was holding out for my hero. I just wanted a guy, the one guy to do the opposite of what everyone else had done. I wanted that one who tells me I am pretty, brings me flowers, and is proud to be with me. I wanted someone to show me what a knight is and that he can be a gentleman. The one person who makes me feels special, always doing something extraordinary and the unexpected. The one that makes me feel and know I am significant.

On January 4, 2012, while sitting in Studio B at the AIM dance studio, a man walked into the room wanting to sign up for the 90 day challenge. He had come to learn about losing weight effectively and taking Zumba dance lessons. His name is Keith Curley, the quiet, small in stature, yet tall in elegance, blue-eyed, fair haired gentleman, who stands as tall as a giant with his character and soars on the shoulders of greatness with kindness and integrity. At the moment he said hello, his voice was so recognizable to me. His voice created a resonance within me. I continued to be drawn to his familiar voice, every time he subsequently entered the studio.

Keith joined our weight loss group and became a regular fixture at AIM's Zumba, then began joining me and my peeps down at St. Basil's and St. Mary's. He originally was the only fellow in the room and would slip in to the back, do his hour of fitness dancing and then just as easily slip out. However, as time went on, I noticed that he seemed to linger around more and be looking in my direction. I probably noticed it, because the same thing was happening with me too. We became friends on Facebook, and started chatting back and forth via email. The smiles at Zumba turned into hugs of hello and goodbye and our simple chit chat evolved into conversations. Eventually, I got brave enough to ask him to go for a walk with me. It took him six months to say yes, but finally we ended up on our first walking excursion on Sunday, September 30, 2012.

Keith had also begun to join us on Saturday mornings at Boot Camp with Gladys Knier, my *Shape Up Brantford* partner. In fact, according to Keith, it was then when he finally admitted to himself, *"I'm hooked."* One Saturday morning, I was dancing like a gazelle jumping through the air during the running warm-up. He kept laughing so hard at me, as I was in my own little world and totally oblivious to anyone else in the room, jumping through the air and attempting to fly while singing. Keith told me that is the morning when I stole his heart.

Every woman in the world waits for *The Look*. We all talk about it, that look a man gives that says he is afraid that if he leaves, he may never see you again. We search to finally see *that look*, the one where you finally see the feelings in your heart staring back at you. I never experienced that look. I've seen it in other couples where they look at one another, I've seen it acted out in movies, I've read about it in novels, but I have never known it. I have wished for it, and perhaps thought that I may have seen a glimmer of it in others, yet I was always wrong. I never saw the look -- the look of love. I started to see that in Keith early on. I knew he liked me, but it wasn't lust, it wasn't about anything other than,

"This man really cares for me." It was in his smile when he saw me and his eyes when I looked back at him. It was in his cautious flirting of calling me "cutie" and telling me how he couldn't get past my eyes. He was very careful as he put his hands on my shoulders, opening the door for me, always being chivalrous long before we had even held hands. There was this little boy excitement in his texts and phone calls, or a giggle from him as he would innocently tell me that he was talking about me at work, becoming a never ending subject.

Keith has asked me not to put too much about him in this book as this is about me and my story. I won't get into too many details of the love story, as Keith has specifically asked me to keep that between us. I understand but he has given me approval for a sequel. I would be remiss to my own plight and my readers, however, if I didn't at least introduce them to the hero of the story. He is thirteen years older than I but exudes youthful exuberance. With his very fit physique and forever smiling face, nobody would be any the wiser that we are not the same age. We are known as the cute couple with matching muscular legs. We call ourselves "Team KEJO." We behave like two sixteen year olds; always holding hands, always kissing, always playing. We are overly passionate and while we have a relationship of laughter, music and dance, two people this passionate are also bound to have impassioned arguments, but we love making up!

I had been single for a long time and have never known the joy of any romance or relationship that was of any quality or substance. I did not know what it is like to be really married, or really have a boyfriend or really know a partnership. I was never given the opportunity. So, ours has been a learning process with me as the very willing pupil.

Keith too has had his own painful moments and recovered from losses and life's altering twists and turns. We were both put in one another's paths to fully realize our true worth and to foster each other's dreams so that with support they become reality. For my entire life, I dreamed about him, I dreamed of finding him and now we live the dream together. His heart is one filled with softness that echoes through his suave demeanour and genuine nice guy characteristics. He lights up a room when people he knows see him and he's always greeted by everyone with the same responsive smiles of others being really happy to see him. I rejoice in the fact that women want to hug him and men are always shaking his hand, high-fiving him or putting their hands on his shoulders. He takes pride in his appearance and while he's generally sporting nice clothes and cleaning up nicely, he is never afraid to muck in and get dirty. He's one of those guys that can do everything and do it well.

Keith has loved me so much and shown me just what it means to really care for someone. He may have once been the quiet guy in the corner; but now he stands beside me and protectively behind me. At the beginning of this chapter, I talked about his voice. I soon realized as I began dating Keith who the voice was. It became clear the first time he said, *"I love you."* I knew where I had heard that voice before. It was HIS voice I heard in my dreams, his voice I heard in my prayers and it was his voice that I heard in the wind at App's Mill. As soon as his voice said those three little words I knew he was my chosen one. I had spent my whole life looking for him and I will now spend the rest of my life looking at him.

In May, 2013, Keith took me to his work's year end gala at Bingemans Banquet Centre, a black tie affair. We were both decked out to the nines. Keith calmly said to me as he held the door open for my entrance, *"Thirty years later, your date has brought you to the prom."* Keith Curley is my actualization of the reasons I could not and would not settle in my past. Inside I just knew there was better. He's my better.

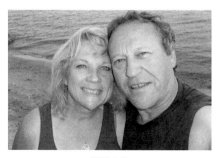

KEJO

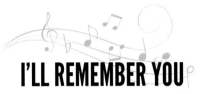

I'LL REMEMBER YOU

I've Left the Building -- Until We Meet Again,
May God Bless You, Adios

It is May 2014. I am sitting on my red lawn chair at Loni's Lookout overlooking the dam in Paris. The sun is warm, the water is cresting over the top and I am flopped in my chair re-reading the book, *Eat Pray Love*. It is this book which inspires me to write my own. I have my tape recorder with me as I recall my journey. I am in a melancholy state and feeling restless. I begin to daydream, going back to a time just before my journey began. I have an almost out-of-body experience as I see my former self sitting exactly where I am, slouched into the red chair, gazing aimlessly with a forlorn look of desperate loss. A short blonde-haired woman walks past the former me, dressed in a familiar outfit of a turquoise tank top, black shorts and black and white flip flops.

The woman walks past and stops to look at me. I seem to be caught in a trance. I turn to look at this woman with my infamous indifferent acknowledgement which turns into an inquisitive double take rubber neck turn. The woman moves about four feet from me and stares straight across to the other side, watching a crane frolic on the rocks. I look at her with a furrowed brow, staring at her with an almost forbidden recognition acceptance of who I am seeing. The blonde continues to stare straight and sputters, *"Nice day, eh?"* I chillingly reply, "Yes, the water is beautiful. I come here a lot!" *"Me too,"* she giggles, *"This is my sanctuary."* Then I look directly at her as I turn around in my chair. With my mouth agape, I question,

"Are you -- I know you. I've seen you before; you're ME twenty years ago." The woman gives a gentle verbal scoff and replies, *"No, Joan, I'm you in two years."* My eyes come out of my head, "That's impossible; you're so youthful and thin." She reassures me yet again, *"Joan, I'm YOU in two years."* My eyes well up, my bottom lip quivers and I begin to tremble as the woman comes near me, and plops down happily on the grass. Her recognizable crooked smile evolves into an almost *To Be or Not to Be* type of soliloquy:

"Just sit right back and you'll hear a tale, a tale of a fateful trip. What a journey you are going on. It is so EPIC! There is so much excitement coming. It's a never-ending kaleidoscope. Your entire landscape is about to change. You are so lucky to have this all ahead of you. I'm actually envious, as this is just beginning for you. That makes me smile. You are going to lose a whole lot of weight. There's no end in sight for the actual number but I can tell you this, it will be substantial. You're going to get healthy Joan. Your body is going to heal. The illnesses will stop. You will conquer the demons and your food addiction. Your weight loss is going to turn into a revolution. The wave is about to hit; ride it with gusto! Embrace every nuance, and get healthy. Oh, Kiddo, please, more than anything, get healthy. You are going to learn about foods you never consumed. You will embrace Waldorf salads and put fruit and nuts into bowls of leafy lettuce. You will embrace the education of making healthier and sane food choices. Your body will be free!"

"You will get perky and spunky and yes you will love yourself again. You will have a love affair with yourself. You will document this love in 'selfies'. You will dance the tarantella. You are going to have fun, learn to flirt again, be playful, gain confidence, and conquer the illnesses that are invading your body. You are going to give yourself the gift of life and forgive. Yes kiddo, you're going to learn to forgive. You will tell your story and then file it under 'No Longer Relevant, Time to Let Go.' You searched your whole life for that special one. Look in the mirror girl; YOU are the one. Look at you sitting here bellyaching. Freaking STOP IT. Disengage, pull the plug. I see the look on your face; I know you are in disbelief. I'm here to tell you, your life is about to change. You DO want it to change right? I see the depth within your eyes; I KNOW you want it to change, so

bloody change it. If you want your life to change, then do something about it and change it. I need to instil in you from this day forward: there is a greater force than you steering this boat. You are just the person standing in the vessel. A power greater than you and me is the captain on this ship. You need to hold on and be prepared for one hell of a ride!"

"There's a message I am bringing, which needs to be the fire under your feet. NEVER GIVE UP. I am here to tell you a story of hope, a tale of success and an adventure of serenity and happiness. What is coming is going to be so worth it. Every tear you cry is going to be the river you walk by along the path. What you feel today will be a once trodden laneway. Stop looking in the rear view mirror. Your past is there. You must turn your sights forward to the windshield and see the amazing scenery of your life ahead of you. The rear view mirror will grow distant and as you move forward all of it must remain in the past, just like your once fat behind. Take a breath, take one final glimpse behind you right now and then say goodbye. The adventure that is coming is going change your life completely. You will be afraid. NEVER GIVE UP!"

"This may sound frightening but most of those who are presently in your life will not be around for very much longer. It will shock you; they will be with you at the onset but will fall off as the success mounts. You will lose friends and this will happen quickly. This will scare and create fear within you. The demons will taunt you and cause you to question everything about yourself. They will advance with fierce determination as they try to break you. NEVER GIVE UP!"

"It is going to be a one sided vicious battle. You are going to be faced with the cruelest of attacks, and your circle of friends will not be reliable enough to have your back. NEVER GIVE UP!"

"The hatred will be churned into your greatest resolve as you embrace the resurgence of a brand new life and a new you. NEVER GIVE UP!"

"It won't be easy. From the pit of your present despair, you will have a historic Cheshire Cat smile awakening. You will succeed. You will take on a new horizon as the care of yourself and BJ will become prolific. Oh, BJ, he's going to be remarkably proud of you

as he shows you off to his friends. You will not recognize yourself; nobody will. The way in which you carry yourself will be the most obvious change as the outpouring of self confidence begins to empower you. Your head and shoulders will rise with the corners of your mouth. You will know inner peace and serenity. You will succeed. NEVER GIVE UP!"

"You are going to be tested like you have never known. You are going to prove to your supporters that you are strong and their belief in you will be the boulevard of dreams comes true. It will be all worth it in the end. You will have physical injuries. You will have stresses. NEVER GIVE UP!"

"Keep your eye on the prize of saving BJ's mom. Please trust me, kiddo, the pay offs will be so fulfilling that you will come to embrace the new you with confidence, love, respect and ultimate self appreciation. NEVER GIVE UP!"

"Remember when you used to hide away and eat when you were a teen? You will find yourself now fit, as you walk daily and cycle through the pathways at Mount Hope Cemetery giving thanks to God. You will find spiritual awakening in the back pew of St. Basil's Church as you form new friendships with the parishioners and clergy while cementing your deep relationship with Christ. Walking along the banks of Webster's Falls in Dundas, it will be the last time you cry over the past and turn it into the eraser you need to let it all go. The weight you will take off your ankles will be miniscule to the weight released off your shoulders. As the days turn into weeks, people's inadequacies surface to weaken you; they will actually strengthen you. All that glitters is not gold, but the shine will become brighter around your face as you embrace the new YOU. Walk right through it. Stand tall -- keep walking. NEVER GIVE UP!"

"As the weight drops off, so will the stress. You will find out you are NOT alone -- an army is coming. Let your humour be as it always has been -- your greatest character trait. It gets better. Walk right through it. Soldier on...Walk right through it back to YOU. It gets easier. You will do this. The figure you have longed for will be yours. The love life you only dreamed about is coming. NEVER GIVE UP!"

"You will face the demons in silence as you walk away

and hold your head up, your lips sealed and you will be the victor. Nothing will stop you. NEVER GIVE UP!"

"Walk through it. The rage of negative energy that swirls around will be matched with your new found energy and healthy calories, which will be a blessing as you take it and use it to help propel your journey forward. The divine plan of God's intervention will all make sense. NEVER GIVE UP!"

"New friendships will be created and a place of sanctuary will be molded for you where you will not only get your groove back but will find true happiness. He's coming. It won't happen right away but the journey back to yourself will lead you to finding that special someone. He will mend all of the shattered pieces of your heart and create a new chamber of peace and contentment. NEVER GIVE UP!"

"You will start to dance again, and rekindle a relationship with your feet that will inspire you to new found heights of motivation. As your body gets healthy, new doors will open as you become involved with exhilarating activities. Your now beaten body will unfold into an athletic beacon of strength. You will sign up to support the United Way as you climb almost two thousand stairs at the CN Tower in Toronto in a phenomenal time of 21 minutes and 34 seconds. As you climb that tower you will rejoice in your physical agility and in a moment of solo time on the seventy fifth floor you will encourage yourself to keep going as you tell yourself 'Minnery you are fit. Look at us. We are doing this. Do it Joan, we are freaking doing it!' As you reach the finish line, the tears streaming down your face will be wiped away by a stranger who grabs and hugs you as you loudly bellow, 'Two years ago I was 300 pounds'. NEVER GIVE UP!"

"Get this kiddo -- over the next few years you will walk over ten thousand kilometres. Yes, you heard that right. There is no end in sight of how many more notches you will place on numerous pairs of running shoes. You will take part in your first five kilometre run at the Brant Fit Fest, an event you will spearhead. NEVER GIVE UP!"

"A whole revolution will take place. A chick named Heather Cardle will come into your life that will be armed with a camera, as she chronicles your milestones in photographs. You will shed one half of yourself in more ways than one. You will lose twelve dress

sizes and an entire shoe size as your body melts as you go through insurmountable amounts of coats, sweaters, pants, boots, tops, socks, bras and undies, and 4 umbrellas! NEVER GIVE UP!"

"Oh kiddo, the rewards that are coming for you! None sweeter than that of the closure you will get when you stand atop the rock at App's Mill and shout to the sky that you forgive those that have wounded you. As you shout to the wilderness, you will be so overcome that you will be forced into a crouched position with an emotional outburst. You will smile as you cry out, 'I'm free at last. Thank God Almighty, I'm free at last!' NEVER GIVE UP!"

"Your Hollywood ending is coming. This is the life you have always dreamed about. It is the finale you envisioned as you ride off into the sunset with the credits of gratitude rising up on the screen. Your star will be the light around you as you become your own Academy Award; your journey will be the canvass for your acceptance speech, but first -- you need to get up off your fat butt, stop the insanity and get moving."

We are both now standing up cheering and embracing. I nod my head but cannot open my mouth. I am completely dumbfounded. She grabs hold of me and squeezes my face *"Rejoice in the triumphs and celebrate all of the good that has come and how far WE have travelled together. WE DID THIS TOGETHER. She, You, Me, Us -- TOGETHER. Yes, find the core for why we're here and focus on THAT. Happiness comes with a price but one that is greatly paid in full with health, a happier heart and a love so profound and unique; nothing can equal its value."*

She pauses and takes my hand. *"The albatross is defeated. We slew the dragon and WON. We did it, kiddo, we bloody did it."* I start to cry happiness. *"Who you are today will never leave you. It will always be a part of you. Always know you are never alone. I am here for you to pull you forward. I am 'weighting' for you on the other side."* She kisses me. Still transfixed, I watch her skip away, noticing she has the strongest calf muscles I have ever seen on a woman.

I wake up from my daydream giggling with two very wet cheeks. I stand up, I look across the water. The crane has now flown off but the water continues to crest over the dam. A train approaches overhead and passes along the bridge. I watch it travel and keep my eyes glued on the last car until it is out of sight. I pack up my chair, put my belongings back into my knapsack and head down the hill. In a few hours I'll be teaching Zumba with Keith in the front row. *"She was right. Nothing is as it was, and I wouldn't trade ANY of it for all the jumpsuits in Memphis."*

As I am about to get into my van, the blonde woman appears once more at my perch at Loni's Lookout. She is waving frantically at me. She happily shouts down to me. *"Kiddo, there's one more thing. It's vitally important, perhaps the greatest advice I can give you -- when someone asks you to pose in a red corset -- DO IT!!!"*

The dancing elephant sings. The blimp smiles. I have walked my way back to me...

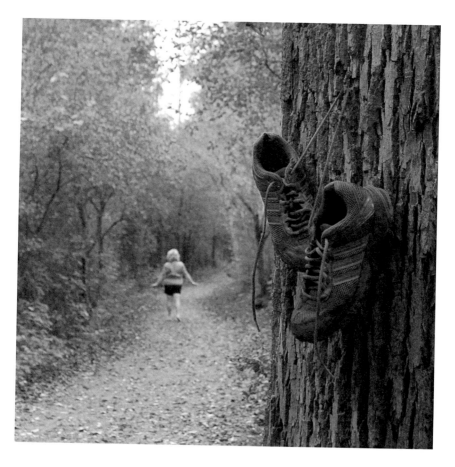